Praise for

No GuessWork and **Dr. Rameck Hunt**

"This book will change your life forever. The reason Dr. Hunt has done so well in his weight management clinic is because No GuessWork works!"
—Sampson Davis, MD, FACEP, *New York Times* best-selling author and emergency medicine physician

"No GuessWork is a game changer! No more confusion. Dr. Hunt lays out the science in an easy-to-follow plan that will help you get to a healthier weight that lasts a lifetime."
—George Jenkins, DMD, MHA, *New York Times* best-selling author and Assistant Dean of Access, Equity and Inclusion at Columbia Dental School

"Dr. Hunt is one of the leading obesity experts who delivers trustworthy information. He discussed one of the most important ingredients of treating obesity, behavioral modification, by discussing mindfulness and motivational interviewing techniques. Readers will pass this book on to their friends and then to their friends and so on. It's just that good and just that important of a book on achieving a healthy lifestyle."
—Camille Archer, MD, psychiatrist

The NO GUESSWORK Diet

Discover Your Carb Number For **Swift, Healthy,** and **Sustainable Weight Loss**

Rameck Hunt, MD, FACP

Published by No GuessWork, LLC

This is a work of prescriptive nonfiction. The events and conversations in this book have been set down to the best of the author's ability, although some names have been changed to protect the privacy of individuals. This book contains supplemental advice and information related to healthcare. This book is not meant in any way to be the source of diagnosis or treatment of any medical or mental health condition. You should always seek the advice of your healthcare provider. Never disregard your healthcare provider's advice or delay seeking medical attention as a result of something you read in this book. This author disclaims liability for any medical outcomes that may result from the use of any information in this book.

For more information: info@noguesswork.com

First edition June 2020

Contributing writer, Lisa Frazier Page
Edited by Anne Cole Norman

Cover design by Stephanie Hannus
Cover photo by Valeria Boltneva
Interior design by David Provolo

ISBN 978-1-7348897-0-3 (paperback)
ISBN 978-1-7348897-3-4 (hardcover)
ISBN 978-1-7348897-1-0 (ebook)

www.noguesswork.com
www.drrameckhunt.com

No GuessWork, LLC

Dedication

This book is dedicated to all those who have struggled with obesity and obesity associated health conditions. I have been so inspired by you, and seeing your success gives me so much hope that we will finally overcome this disease.

TABLE OF CONTENTS

Preface

I was listening to my favorite radio show one morning in 2018 and heard one of the co-hosts fat-shaming people. "Fat people are just lazy," he said. "They eat too much and are just not disciplined enough to do anything about it." The comments stunned me, even coming from this particular host, who has made a name for himself by being controversial and opinionated. I'm a fan of the show, but on this matter, he was flat wrong.

My instinct to do something kicked in, and I texted a friend, who happens to be his co-host, and shared some facts to relay to him to get him to stop the fat-shaming. Surprisingly, she went a step further and invited me to their show to discuss obesity. I knew that the host's views about obesity reflect the way that many people who have never struggled with the disease think. Unfortunately, many who struggle with obesity think that way, as well. And so do many doctors. Like many people, I'd never even considered obesity a disease until I began studying it. Given the radio host's controversial views, I also knew that if I accepted his invitation, the conversation would be lively. But this was my opportunity to set the record straight. Since I'm not only a medical doctor but also an obesity medicine specialist who founded an obesity clinic through Penn Medicine Princeton Health in New Jersey, I was the expert. And as I saw it, I really wouldn't be speaking just to the radio host but to the millions of people out there who listen to him every day, including only God knows how many others who share his misguided views on obesity. So, I willingly took the bait.

I showed up, armed with diagrams and graphs, illustrating that obesity is a disease and how the body resists when a person tries to lose weight. I explained that obesity is not the fault of the person who is struggling because the body of a person with obesity literally fights off any attempt to shed the weight. My friend listened and seemed intrigued by what she learned. But the other two co-hosts, particularly the one determined to be my nemesis on this issue, refused to budge on their positions. They just kept circling back to their main talking points: obesity is a matter of willpower; it's all about choices; and people just need to eat less and exercise more. That is, after all, what we as a society have been taught about obesity and weight loss. But science has proven that the battle against obesity is more complex than that. In this book, I help you to see the bigger picture. I help you to understand the forces fighting against you. But most importantly, I give you the weapons to win this battle against obesity for good.

Introduction

You've heard it many times before: the way to lose weight is to eat less and exercise more. Right? It's all about willpower and discipline, we've been told.

Well, not exactly.

I'm a medical doctor, and before I began studying obesity and practicing obesity medicine, I thought that way, too. Quite frankly, changing that mindset is part of the reason I am writing this book. Much of what we as a nation have been fed through the years about how to eat and how to lose weight has been based on lies. The truth is people can eat until they are satisfied if they understand *what* to eat. That is far more important than portion size. And people tend to think that "move more" means going to the gym or signing up for a killer boot camp-style workout regimen, when there are much more simple ways to maximize their activity throughout the day to get the same or even greater benefits.

This book introduces my No Guesswork (NGW) Plan, which will teach you exactly what you need to know to embark on a lifetime of good health and wellness. For too long, we have been misinformed about which foods make us gain weight, and which don't. We've been cutting calories and starving ourselves to shed the pounds, only to gain the weight back again, wondering if we have to be hungry all the time in order to maintain a healthy weight. We've had to guess—is there any diet out there that will help me stay slim and healthy for good? My plan takes the guesswork out of healthy living, and it will change your life. No more diet confusion, no more shooting in the dark. You will lose weight, but most importantly, you will learn how to keep the weight off for life.

Obesity is epidemic in this country. About 42.4 percent of adults in the United States have obesity, according to a 2017-2018 report from the Centers for Disease Control and Prevention. The problem is most severe among African Americans (49.6 percent) and Hispanics (44.8 percent). The prevalence of obesity in children ages 2 to 19 is 18.5 percent, affecting about 13.7 million children and adolescents. Predictions are that the obesity crisis will continue to grow. To change, Americans need to understand how we got here and how to get out. My book offers both.

The No Guesswork Plan is more than the typical lose-weight-quick scheme. Here, you will get:

- A simple-to-follow low-carb plan that enables you to eat ample protein and fat-filled meals and snacks that fill you up and keep you from being hungry.
- A customized number that tells you the maximum number of carb grams that you as an individual can eat each day and still lose weight.
- A three-phase plan, starting with Phase One, in which you find and test your customized number; Phase Two, in which you make a few tweaks after losing ten percent of your body weight; and Phase Three (Maintenance, the most important phase), where you learn how to transition into a low-carb, Mediterranean meal plan that will help you maintain your weight loss with a heart-healthy diet for the rest of your life.
- Inspirational stories of patients who have lost weight—and kept it off—on No Guesswork.

In addition, my book offers:

- A breakdown of the low-fat lies that helped create the obesity epidemic.
- An easy-to-understand explanation of the science that supports my program.
- The understanding that obesity is a disease.
- Encouragement that you can defeat it.

My goal is to change the perception of how Americans think about people with obesity. I want the fat-shaming to stop, even among those who live with obesity. I want to educate people that obesity is a real disease with real causes and consequences. When I say that obesity is not the fault of the people who are struggling with it, I'm not just making excuses for them. Science has proven the *battle of the brain* that they fight every day, and I explain that within these pages. Yes, they have some responsibility in making better choices, just as a person who suffers from, say, diabetes or high blood pressure. But for too long people have not been told the truth about what the best choices are.

I wrote this book to tell you the truth and to provide you at last with the No Guesswork Plan for weight loss and healthy living. If you need inspiration and coaching, you will find it here, too. I've been told that diet books are just supposed to tell you what to do, and that's it. We just want a quick fix, I've heard repeatedly. There is certainly no shortage of those kinds of books out there. You read them, lose weight, and then gain it right back. Why? Perhaps we didn't know how the food we were eating affected us. Perhaps we didn't know that the foods we eat ignite a swirl of hormones and cravings in our bodies, or that cutting calories would slow our metabolism. I am here to arm you with the knowledge you need to change your eating habits for good. I dare you to trust your intelligence, to trust that you not only want to lose weight but that you want to know the hidden truth about what really causes us to gain weight. When you know the truth, you can make different and better choices.

My clinic at Penn Medicine Princeton Health focuses on weight maintenance because that is truly the goal: to help our patients achieve a healthy weight and maintain it for the rest of their lives. Our team has helped hundreds of people lose hundreds of pounds. We are so full that we cannot accept any new patients. But I lay out my plan for you in this book. I know it works. If you're ready to change your life, this is the book for you.

AUTHOR'S NOTE — PEOPLE-FIRST LANGUAGE

People-first language emphasizes the person instead of his/her disability or disease. By doing so, the disability/disease is no longer the focus of a person, making the terminology person-centered, and not disease- or disability-centered. Therefore, we will be using people-first language throughout this book, particularly in regards to overweight and obesity. In this book overweight and obesity is regarded as a medical issue, not a descriptor of a person. So, you will see language, such as "the person has overweight" or "the person has obesity" (we won't use "the person is obese" in describing a person). This may sound strange and unfamiliar at first glance, but as mentioned, we are using those words as nouns (i.e. as medical conditions), not as an adjective that describes a person, such as the adjective cheerful. There will be a few times in the book where I will purposely not use people-first language, and that will be in context of the sentence in which it is being used or a quote from someone.

CHAPTER ONE

A Life-Altering Question

I didn't set out to become an obesity doctor. After graduating from medical school, I had just worked with two of my best friends on our first book, *The Pact: Three Young Men Make a Promise and Fulfill a Dream*, which details our journey from poor, troubled youths in Newark, New Jersey, to becoming doctors (two medical doctors and a dentist). The book debuted on *The New York Times* bestseller list and stayed there for several weeks. We followed up with two more bestselling books. The three of us were (and still are) traveling the country giving inspirational talks and doing some exciting community work though our non-profit organization, The Three Doctors Foundation. I had found my calling in life. Inspiring people from blighted communities, in particular, and communities across the country, in general, especially the youth, became part of my mission. My medical career as an internal medicine specialist was burgeoning, as well. I had a thriving medical practice and a purposeful mission, so I thought my career journey was complete. All the things I wanted professionally in life, I'd accomplished. All the things I was passionate about doing, I was doing. Besides having a wife and children, I couldn't imagine anything else that could so ignite my passion, much less fit into my schedule.

Then came Sharon.

The Inspiration

Sharon was a 45-year-old wife and mother of three when she became my patient around 2007, along with her husband. She was a sweet, soft-spoken woman with a calming presence. She had the gift of making anyone in her presence somehow just feel relaxed.

Back then, she already had at least 100 pounds in excess weight. Her list of medical problems included hypertension and high cholesterol, and I later diagnosed her with sleep apnea. She was really interested in getting healthy and wanted to get off the blood pressure medication she was taking. I told her the best thing she could do was to lose weight. Of course, she knew that, but she was looking to me for guidance. Unfortunately, all I had in my tool box then were four words: eat less, move more. That's pretty typical. One of the things most doctors don't do is talk about weight, and when they do, the tools they usually have to offer are the same limited ones I had.

A nationwide study of attitudes and behaviors related to obesity revealed some of the barriers people with obesity face in getting appropriate healthcare. The Awareness Care and Treatment in Obesity Management (ACTION) study, from 2017, found that most people with obesity don't get a medical diagnosis of obesity or a referral for medical care. Just 24 percent of doctors who identified a patient with obesity scheduled a follow-up appointment with the patient to address that issue. The study also found that 82 percent of people with obesity believe their condition is their responsibility alone to handle. The study, which involved 3,000 patients, 600 health care professionals, and 150 employers, is believed to be the first in the United States to examine treatment barriers from the perspective of people living with the disease.

Doctors are generally not trained in medical school to deal with patients' weight issues, so we don't talk about what we don't know. It's easier, I suppose, just to put the blame and responsibility on the patient. However, the health industry is pushing medical professionals to change somewhat. Now, Medicare and many insurance companies require doctors to note on a patient's record if the patient has overweight or obesity. The payers are essentially requiring us doctors to acknowledge the connection between obesity and diseases in a more formal way. The presumption is that such acknowledgement will force doctors to have more substantial conversations with their patients about weight.

I definitely needed to talk to Sharon about her weight. Over time, Sharon gained even more weight. Her blood pressure eventually shot up to dangerous levels, and I was worried. By then, she was going through a divorce, had slipped into depression, and was not taking good care of herself. So, instead of taking her off the blood pressure medicine, as she had long hoped, I had to increase it. Sharon promised to get the pounds off, but for a long time, nothing changed.

Her appointment in the summer of 2010 was different, though. She had gained five pounds just in the three weeks since her previous visit. We were reviewing her bloodwork, and not only was her blood pressure out of control, but she had also developed pre-diabetes. I was deeply concerned about her. I knew she was a mother and that her children meant the world to her. So, when we sat down to discuss the results of her tests, I told her I was concerned about her health. She was taking care of everyone else, but if she didn't get her weight under control, I was worried she might not be around to see them all grow up. I asked about the health of her three kids: "Are your children obese?"

Sharon looked startled and hurt. I hoped she could tell by the tone of my voice that I wasn't trying to be mean, but it didn't matter. She burst into tears, and I immediately wished I could take back my words. For the next few minutes, Sharon sobbed uncontrollably, expressing feelings of deep guilt. What I couldn't have known then was that her son, then about to become an eighth grader, had recently come to her with a heartbreaking concern: He didn't want to feel like the fattest kid in school and wanted to lose weight. My question had brought the pain home to Sharon: she was the one feeding her children, and so not only was she hurting herself, but she was hurting them.

Sharon left my office that day with a quiet determination in her eyes that I had never before seen in her. A few months later, when she returned for her next visit, I was astonished. She had lost a significant amount of weight, and with every visit after that, she just kept getting smaller. Over about two years, she lost 127 pounds, and she did it on her own, mostly by following a low-calorie program that required her to track her food intake and limit her calories. She cut out sweets and other refined carbohydrates. She also began walking faithfully with a friend around a track near her house several times a week.

I told Sharon how proud I was of her and encouraged her every step of the way. It was one of my proudest days as a physician when I took her off all of the blood pressure medications, except for a mild water pill that kept her legs from swelling during the hot and humid summer months. Sharon not only would keep the weight off, but she would go on to run in 5K races and even a half-marathon. She amazed me, but I knew I couldn't take much credit for her success. She says I inspired her and that she might never have discovered the healthy person she became without that inspiration. But truly, she inspired me.

In seeing her success and how much it affected her health for the better, I was determined to find out more about the science of obesity so I could better help my patients. In the early years of my medical career, I'd never even thought much about how to treat obesity, beyond the cursory "eat less, move more" advice I gave to patients with overweight or obesity. It was all we had been taught in medical school. As an internal medicine specialist for Penn Medicine Princeton Health Systems, I treated lots of patients struggling with weight-related illnesses, such as diabetes, heart disease, and high blood pressure, the so-called triple threat, as we coined it in residency. Somehow, though, I knew the "eat less, move more" mantra just wasn't quite right. I wanted to be able to do more than just *tell* my patients to lose weight; I wanted to show them how. The timing was fortuitous, too, because the idea that I should find my niche in medicine had begun percolating in my head. Working in internal medicine was starting to feel a bit like being a "jack of all trades, master of none," as the old saying goes. I'd also grown tired of prescribing pills and ordering expensive medical procedures to treat health problems that could be relieved by weight loss. Sharon was the rare patient who had managed to change her entire health status with dramatic weight loss. Maybe with my guidance, other patients could do it, too.

It's Not Your Fault

Curious about what resources were out there, I turned to Google to find an organization for doctors who specialize in treating people who have obesity. The American Society of Bariatric Physicians (now called the Obesity Medicine Association) popped up. I read everything I could find and learned that the organization was having a conference in the near future. Just a couple of months later, in September 2014, I joined the estimated 600 physicians at the conference in Austin, Texas. Many of the doctors there had been practicing internal medicine, like me, and I felt at home among them. They shared the camaraderie of a group with inside knowledge about an epidemic not widely understood in the broader medical community. They talked about obesity as a disease, without assigning any more blame to the one afflicted than a doctor would do to a patient suffering from any other disease. Yes, obesity is a disease, and it has pathways that cause it (termed pathophysiology), and those pathways have very little to do with a person's willpower (as I will explain in the next chapter). Not only that, but obesity has many factors that contribute to the disease, such as: genetics (including gut hormones and your metabolism, something called metabolic adaptation), your surroundings, medications, your endocrine and immune systems, and behavior. Genetics is involved in every aspect of life, so it's the biggest factor of all.

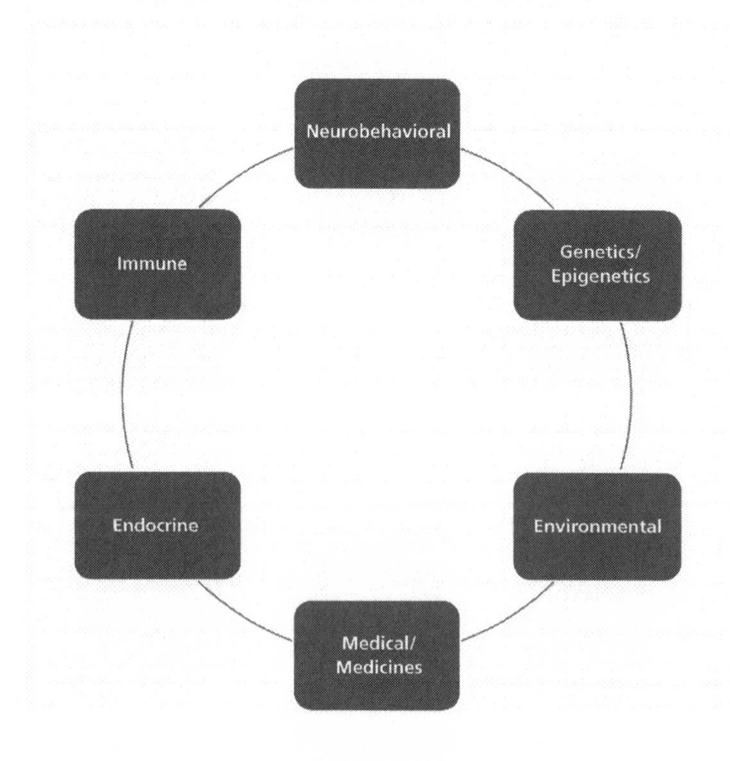

So we have to think about and address all of these factors to effectively treat obesity. Evidence of how important a role genetics play in obesity is show in twin studies. These studies show that identical twins are virtually the same weight (and height) throughout life, while in non-identical twins, weight (and height) varies. This demonstrates how powerful our genes are in regulating our metabolism and the hormones involved in weight control. The good news is, although every individual does it a little differently, we know a lot about how your body (i.e. your genes) does this. And because of this we have a much better handle on fighting obesity.

GENETICS PLAY A MAJOR ROLE IN OBESITY

Non-identical/Fraternal (Dizygotic) Twins

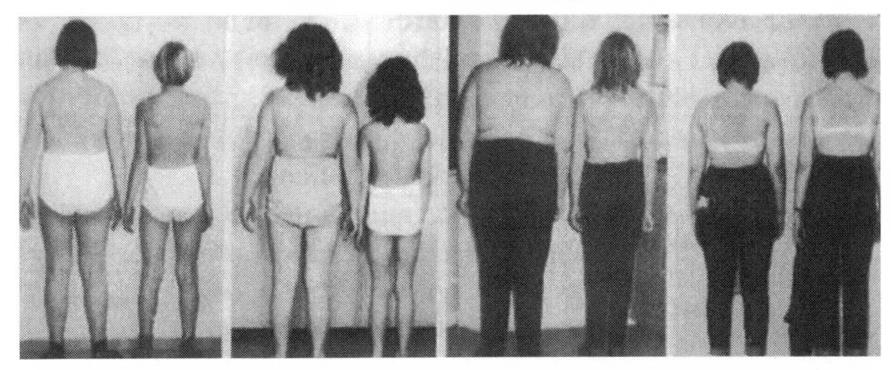

Identical (Monozygotic)Twins

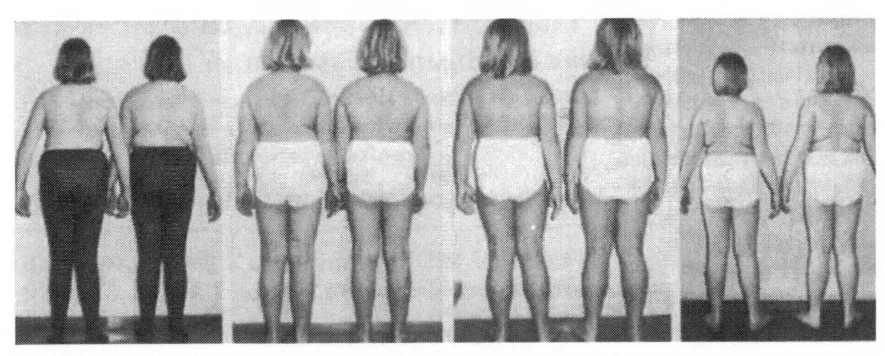

This was all new to me. Like most people, I'd always thought of obesity as a factor of willpower and discipline, which is why I was so shocked when a speaker in one of the sessions casually said something like, "We all know obesity is not the patient's fault." Members of the audience nodded in agreement, as if this was common knowledge. I felt like the guy who walks up in the middle of a conversation that everybody else is having. But I quickly became like a new convert at a religious revival that was unveiling life-altering truth. The speaker talked about how hormones in the gut communicate with the brain to control hunger, make you crave certain types of food, and actually fight against the body's efforts to lose weight. When it feels threatened by significant weight loss, your body also can lower your metabolism, making it harder for you to lose more weight and easier for you to regain the weight you lost. That's why the vast majority of people who lose a significant number of pounds gain them back in a short amount of time. I soaked up this new information. I wanted to understand more about how this all works and what the scientific community could do to find solutions, short of bariatric surgery, for the many people who are struggling. I'd found a new passion. I wanted to be part of the solution.

At one point during the conference, a group of us went to dinner. I sat next to Dr. Eric Westman, who was the president of the American Society of Bariatric Physicians at that time, and a group of monks, who had traveled several hours to learn from him. Dr. Westman had written a book about a ketogenic (low-carb) diet. The monks had experienced success with his plan and asked if they could join us for dinner. Yes, of course, he said, and I sat there, listening to their conversation. They thanked him and asked him questions to better understand the science behind the low-carb diet. As I sat there listening to their conversation, I thought to myself that the knowledge in that room could be transformative for people struggling with weight loss.

Carbs: The Real Culprit

Most of the individual doctors I met at the conference were proponents of a low-carb lifestyle. This left an impression on me. These were the professionals who treated patients who had obesity all day every day and, as I saw it, they are far more likely to understand what diets work best and why. What I learned from them upset everything I thought I knew about weight loss. For years, I'd been telling my patients to eat a low-fat diet and exercise more. Too much fat makes you fat—that's what we'd all been trained to believe, right? Well, as it turns out, eating fat doesn't make you fat; it can actually help make you thin. Carbohydrates (carbs) are the real culprits; in particular, sugar and refined carbohydrates. I make a point to specifically say sugar and refined carbohydrates because I don't want to make the same mistake those before me made when they blamed everything on one macronutrient, fat.

Carbs make up about half of the typical American diet— about 312 grams of carbs per day in a 2,500-calorie diet. That is far more than most people burn in a day. During the digestive process, carbs are converted into sugar and burned first—before anything else that you eat—for energy. The carbs that are not burned are converted to fat and stored in fat cells. A low-carb diet pushes the body to burn fat *instead* of carbs as the primary source of energy. This fat-burning process can put you in a state called ketosis; thus, some low-carb meal plans are called ketogenic diets. This is a simplistic explanation of a more complex process, but the science made sense to me when I first heard it.

Mind you, I don't want to sound like I'd never heard of a low-carb diet. Low-carb diets aren't new. The Atkins Diet has been around forever, but I'd never paid much attention to its scientific claims. I've never dieted much myself, and I thought Atkins was a fad, like all of the other lose-weight-quick schemes out there, but I would later learn that wasn't the case. At that 2014 conference, I became mesmerized by science that backed up the health benefits of a low-carb diet.

At the time of the conference, a documentary called *Fed Up* had been released just months earlier and was generating much buzz among the physicians. One of the speakers suggested we all watch it. Narrated and produced in part by Katie Couric, the groundbreaking film explores the connection between the proliferation of sugar in the nation's foods and the obesity epidemic, particularly among children. It's of note that in the 1980s almost no kids had Type 2 diabetes, except for very rare case reports, which is why it was called adult-onset diabetes at the time. But by 2015, a total of 193,000 children and adolescents younger than 20 were diagnosed with diabetes, and about 90 to 95 percent of those cases were obesity-related. *Fed Up* points out that one in five (nearly 20 percent) of school-aged children (ages six to nineteen) now have obesity, compared to one in twenty children (5 percent) in the 1970s. The film suggests that the so-called solutions for obesity actually may have helped to make the problem worse. The implication is that the increased sugar, which was added to low-fat foods to improve the taste when the fat was removed, actually made the foods less healthy. And even though fitness club memberships doubled between 1980 and 2000, so did the obesity rate. Between 1977, the start of the low-fat craze, and 2000, the intake of sugar doubled among Americans, as many made the switch to low-fat processed foods. During the same time frame, the obesity rate doubled.

The increase of sugar in American diets has been so alarming that in 2016, the U.S. Food and Drug Administration changed nutrition labels on foods to require a new line for "added sugar" to distinguish between sugar that is in food naturally and sugar added to improve the taste. Researchers from the University of North Carolina found in a detailed study that 60 percent of packaged foods and drinks purchased from American grocery stores—from sauces and soups to fruit juices—have added sugar in some form. The danger is that studies on lab rats have shown that sugar is even more addictive than cocaine. Every child that came of age after 1980 grew up with sugary foods, and sadly, this generation is expected to lead a shorter lifespan than their parents. All the while, we were told fat was the enemy, while sugar and refined carbohydrates were really the culprits. We didn't know how they were affecting our bodies and continued to consume them even as we tried to lose weight. In the late 1970s during U.S. Senate hearings for the first-ever dietary guidelines for the American people, Senator McGovern, chairman of the committee that created the guidelines, was warned that the science wasn't there yet to prove whether the change to a low-fat diet would make us healthier. He responded that we didn't have time to wait for the science; we had to act right away. That turned out to be a deadly mistake.

As I learned more about the obesity epidemic, especially the crisis among our children, I couldn't help thinking about Sharon and her son (as well as her two daughters), whose own struggle with obesity had brought her to tears in my office that day. If I'd had any doubt before about the next phase of my medical career, it was all gone. I would get board-certified in obesity medicine and become part of the solution.

Practicing What I Preached

In the airport on the way home from the conference, fellow doctors encouraged me to start studying right away and to take the test when it was offered a few months later. So, I bought the study materials, paid the $1,000 test fee, and dug in, balancing my studies with my daily medical practice. I also decided to practice what I was learning in real time. As I learned something, my patients learned it, too. Some of my patients included nurses and other staff members at the hospital where I worked; a number of them had excess weight and wanted to shed some pounds. I told them the basics, to reduce their daily intake of carbs below 100 grams (with a target of 75 grams). I also explained that if they kept their carbs even lower, below 50 grams, the body would undoubtedly go into ketosis and weight loss would be quick and assured. I had them keep a food log of their carbs.

Personally, I wanted to know whether a low-carb diet was sustainable and what kinds of issues my patients might face, so I decided to follow a low-carb eating plan, as well. At six feet tall, I usually weighed in at around 220 pounds, which is considered overweight, according to the Body Mass Index scale used by most doctors (even though I never really thought of myself as overweight, the irony is that I was just 0.17 pounds from developing obesity). But I wanted to get back down to a comfortable weight, between 190 to 200 pounds. In college, I had been a thin kid, about 180 pounds or so, and had slowly gained forty pounds through medical school, residency, and my early days of practicing medicine. Before starting the low-carb diet, I'd even gotten up to 230 pounds. I'm pretty active, which is generally defined as getting at least 10,000 steps a day. At the time, I played basketball once or twice a week and worked out at least three to four times a week. Over the next eight months to a year, I lost twenty pounds by monitoring my carb intake! Losing those twenty pounds made me feel and look so much better, and the process wasn't nearly as difficult as I'd imagined. I love to eat, and I found that with a low-carb eating plan, I could still eat enough to feel satisfied and at the same time continue to enjoy many of my favorite foods. I just had to tailor my food choices a bit. As long as I kept my low-carb snacks around and ate enough of the right foods at mealtime, I wasn't hungry.

The colleagues I was treating also began to lose weight. Their level of activity ranged from person to person; some were very active, while others were barely active at all. But regardless of how active they were, those who stuck to a low-carb meal plan lost weight, while those who faltered did not.

Let's talk about exercise for a moment. Another myth in the weight loss industry is that regular exercise is the key to weight loss. While it is true that exercise helps to burn calories, an hour of intense working out in the gym most likely isn't even enough to burn off the calories you ate at breakfast. The truth is that 80 percent of weight loss is determined by what you put in your mouth. That's right—what you eat determines by far whether or not you will lose weight. For example, I had knee surgery in April 2017 and suddenly could no longer play basketball or exercise, as I usually did. I found that super frustrating and worried that I might begin to pick up weight. However, because I stuck to my low-carb diet, just slightly reducing the number of carbs I was consuming, I actually *lost* an additional ten pounds over the month that I could not move at all.

Now, don't get me wrong. I don't want anybody misinterpreting this, telling folks that "Dr. Hunt says you don't have to exercise!" That is *not* what I'm saying. Exercise is important for medical reasons, including weight loss, and I highly recommend it to all of my patients. But if weight loss is your primary goal, your primary focus has to be on making good food choices first—foods that are low in carbs and high in proteins and fats—yes, fat! I will talk more in detail about that later. I also will discuss later how to build more physical activity into your daily routines, which actually may be more beneficial than a half-hour or hour-long workout at the gym a few times a week.

Since losing those thirty pounds, I have been able to maintain a low-carb lifestyle and a weight of 190 pounds, a healthy weight for me. I also obtained my certification as a bariatrician (whose title later changed to obesity medicine specialist) at the beginning of 2015. As my co-workers and patients began showing dramatic weight loss results, word quickly spread. New patients began seeking me out for help. Initially, I was not only their medical doctor, but also their therapist, nutritionist, and anything else they needed to be successful—and they were very successful.

The Hunt Theory

During the first year of helping more and more patients to lose weight, I began to notice a peculiar thing: my patients were consuming different amounts of carbs, though all less than 100 grams, and still losing on average one to two pounds a week. I began to think: maybe it wasn't necessary for everyone to get their carbs down to the standard ketosis range, the theory that Dr. Atkins popularized, to experience consistent weight loss. That's when I began to develop what I call "the Hunt theory," the notion that it was possible to develop a personalized plan to help each patient discover his or her "carb number," the maximum number of carb grams a person can eat in a day and lose at least one to two pounds a week. I developed a plan that helped each of my patients find his or her carb number, and it worked! My plan is not considered a ketogenic diet because some patients don't have to reduce their carbohydrates to the point of what is considered the ketogenic range to lose weight. Over time, I've refined the process, but the premise remains the same: that a "Weight Loss Carb Number" and a different "Weight Maintenance Carb Number" exist for each of us because our bodies burn fat and operate differently. Imagine that—we're not all the same! People with a more active metabolism can eat more carbs than a person whose metabolism is slower and still lose weight. But both can be successful losing weight and maintaining their weight loss. Once you know your number, weight loss is sure, swift, and above all, healthy.

By the time I went to hospital administrators at Princeton Medical Center to ask for more resources in 2015, they had heard about my successes with treating patients who had overweight and obesity. A few of the top administrators at the hospital had joined my program. Again, timing worked in my favor. Unbeknownst to me, the hospital's leaders already were considering opening a specialized center for bariatrics, and they had three surgeons on board. But they needed a medical doctor who specialized in obesity to treat patients who did not need or want to go the surgical route. It all came together, and I became the founder and medical director of Princeton Medical Center's Weight Management Program, located within the Center for Bariatric Surgery and Metabolic Medicine. I established the program's protocol, based on the four pillars of weight loss:

- Nutrition. We would teach about the benefits of a low-carb diet.
- Behavior Modification. We would use a process called "motivational interviewing," where a practitioner helps patients to understand on their own why they are eating the way they are eating and help them make the needed adjustments to change.
- Physical Activity. We would encourage them to move their bodies more by exercising and building more movement into their everyday activities.
- Medication and/or Bariatric Surgery. If needed, we would prescribe some of the newer, more effective and safe drugs on the market to assist in controlling hunger and cravings. Also, we would refer a qualified patient to a surgeon to consider one of a number of surgical procedures offered for weight loss. To qualify, a patient would have to have a Body Mass Index (BMI) of 40 and a medical description that used to be called "morbidly obese"; the new, more appropriate term is "Class III Obesity." A person with a BMI of 35 (now called Class II Obesity) also qualifies if that person has an associated health condition and has failed medically supervised attempts to lose weight.

Penn Medicine Princeton Health dedicated the necessary resources to my Weight Management Program—a nurse practitioner, therapist, nutritionist, personal trainer, and all the equipment I needed. The same year, 2015, I was honored to be named the New Jersey Hospital Association Healthcare Professional of the Year for my work in both internal medicine and obesity medicine. It was a tremendous personal honor, but I was excited that it opened more opportunities for me to talk about obesity.

The need in this country for specialized attention to obesity is indisputable. An estimated 71 percent of all Americans have either overweight or obesity, according to a Centers for Disease Control and Prevention (CDC) study of overweight/obesity trends from 1988 to 2016. The crisis is even more severe among African Americans, where 71 percent of African American men and 81 percent of African American women has either overweight or obesity, the same study shows. A study by a group of researchers from the Johns Hopkins Bloomberg School of Public Health suggests that if the current trends continue, an astonishing 86 percent of Americans could have overweight or obesity by 2030.

Obesity cuts across all racial and ethnic groups and all income levels. I've treated corporate executives, whose struggle is no different than the indigent patients I've also treated. According to the Centers for Disease Control and Prevention, more than a third of all U.S. adults suffer from a condition known as metabolic syndrome, meaning they have a combination of at least three medical conditions that increase their probability of developing type 2 diabetes, stroke, and heart disease. Those conditions include high blood pressure, high level of triglycerides, low levels of HDL cholesterol (the so-called good cholesterol), high fasting glucose level, and abdominal fat. CDC data shows that between 1988 and 2012, metabolic syndrome increased across every socio-demographic group and so has type 2 diabetes, and these numbers are expected to grow. These conditions and many others are tied to obesity. But there is so much information—and dare I say, misinformation—out there that people don't know what to do. The number of weight loss options and programs available is dizzying, and none of them teaches you a thing about the hard-core science behind why people have obesity and why they haven't been able to keep the weight off. Consider this book as my hand pushing all of that aside. I want you to understand the science in as simple terms as possible, and I want you to have the confidence that you can do this. You *can* lose weight in a healthy way without being hungry. And you can keep it off!

This book will give you the clarity you need to lose weight and manage it for the rest of your life. Best of all, this program is personalized just for you. Many people have told me that the books I've written with my friends as part of The Three Doctors—*The Pact, We Beat the Street* and *The Bond*—made a huge difference in their lives. I truly hope that this book will have the same kind of impact.

CHAPTER TWO

The Fat Truth

The dominant medical and cultural belief about dieting is that fat makes you fat, but the opposite has become abundantly clear: it can actually help you get thinner. So, I think it is important to share a bit of the science behind obesity, as well as some history that might explain why Americans have been slow to embrace a low-carb diet. My hope is that the next two chapters will better explain why I recommend this lifestyle. In turn, you will have a better understanding of why you are doing what you are doing with my No Guesswork (NGW) Plan, which should make it easier for you to stick to this new way of eating and living. As I've said, this journey is not just about weight loss; it's also about weight maintenance, keeping the weight off. If you want a quick fix, yes, you will get results. But if you don't change your lifestyle permanently, you also will end up back at square one. As I always tell my patients, "If you go back to eating the way you were always eating, you will go back to the weight you always were."

Keep in mind that I am trying to do in one chapter what experts—like Dr. Eric Westman, Dr. Stephen Phinney, and Dr. Jeff Volek—did in volumes of published papers and books. Authors Nina Teicholz and Gary Taubes also have dedicated entire books to the topic. So, this is my attempt to highlight the salient points in an easily digestible way. I will make a concerted effort to stay out of the weeds. But if you want to learn more in greater detail, I recommend you read books on the subject by the authors I just mentioned.

The 6 S's

We hear every day about this new diet or that one, and yet Americans are still gaining weight. What people really want to know is, which diet is best? To be honest, many diets work, but for what? Weight loss? Health? Both? Some diets are better than others, and some are more sustainable than others (sustainability is a bit of a trick question, but I'll explain that later). So when I say a low-carb diet is a better diet (i.e. lifelong plan) for most Americans, I mean all of the above. It's what I call the 6 S's: Simple, Safe, Sustainable, Satisfying, Superior (for weight loss) and Sugarless. When compared to other lifestyle changes/diets, a low-carb diet is best for weight loss and best for health, based on blood tests for things like glucose, cholesterol, inflammatory markers, etc. A low-carb diet is more sustainable (it doesn't leave you hungry), and it is safe. I know when many of you think of a low-carb diet, you picture burgers, bacon, and steak, an image that is often linked with the Atkins Diet. That's not at all the low-carb diet I'm talking about; in fact, that's not the Atkins Diet either. A low-carb diet is a colorful diet.

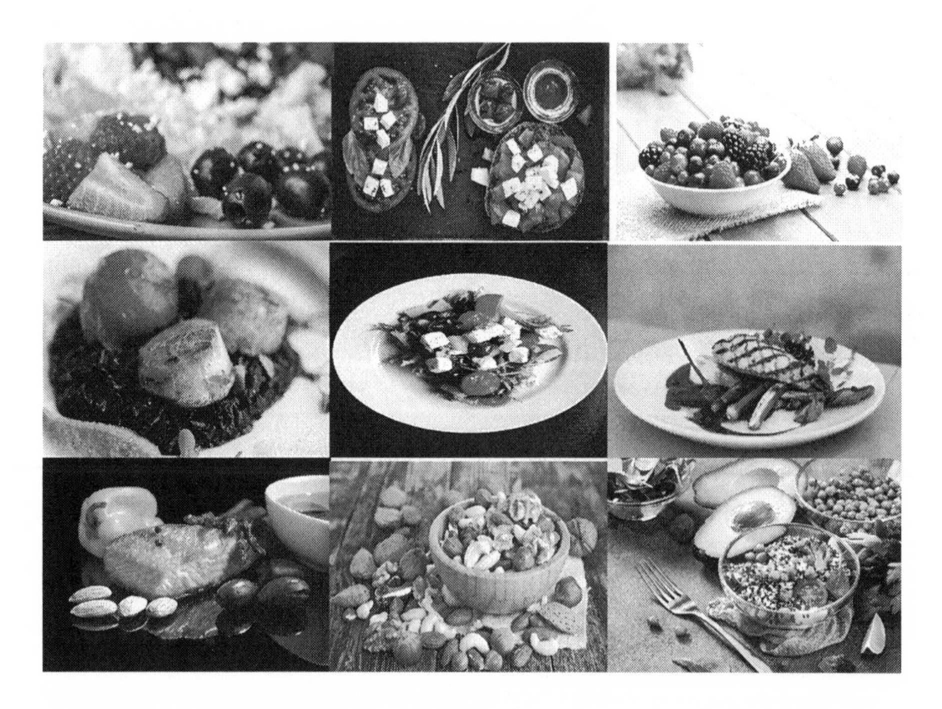

It's similar to how you would envision a whole food, plant-based diet, just with fewer carbs and starches. In fact, the diet I ultimately will recommend for you in this book is a low-carb Mediterranean diet (we just have to get you off the carbs first). Admittedly, I know convincing many of you of this will be a tough feat, given what we have been taught about a healthy diet over the last fifty years. I know, too, how confusing it can be when we hear so much conflicting information about what we should and should not eat.

I was reminded of that recently when a physician friend of mine sent me a text message after watching a popular Netflix documentary about processed food and meat in which one doctor suggested that sugar is not bad and that it's fat that causes health problems, like diabetes. My friend was frustrated. The two of us went back and forth via texts about some of the false claims the physicians in the documentary were making about sugar and carbs. One doctor said that diabetes is not caused by a high-carb diet. Wrong! You don't have to be a doctor to know that if you eat too many carbs, your blood sugar increases and worsens, which can cause type 2 diabetes. Another doctor in the film said that eating fat causes diabetes, not sugar and carbs. Wrong again for the same reason! There's so much misinformation out there. Let me say this now and get it out of the way: Sugar is not good for you, period. It is important to note that sugar is a processed food, and it can be very difficult to produce. The process of getting sugar from sugar cane to the dish on your table is not even close to natural. Plus, sugar has absolutely no nutritional value. No thiamine, no iron, no Vitamin B, no nothing! The last text message from my friend said this: "Well, there are all kinds of doctors out there promoting all kinds of things. It's so difficult for patients who don't understand the science."

Keys to Confusion

My friend is right. The array of conflicting data is even confusing for physicians, who have at least a rudimentary understanding of the science. So I want to point out a couple things. First, to be able to answer definitively, once and for all, the question of which diet formulation works best, researchers would have to lock participants in a simulated society for years – maybe decades — and make them eat a certain diet, monitoring everything they put in their mouths. They would need to track all of their activity and keep detailed records of health-related events (death, stroke, heart attack, cancer, etc.). To take the data one step further, researchers then would have to determine if certain populations (groups based on gender, ethnicity, age, etc.) respond differently to the various diets and whether certain diseases, such as diabetes, respond differently. Clearly, a study like that would cost billions. And I doubt very seriously researchers could find enough healthy subjects (or people with medical issues) willing to spend a good portion of their lives locked in a research lab, eating and drinking only as they are told to do. So scientists have to conduct smaller studies with shorter durations and give expert opinions about what the results of these smaller studies mean. Or, if longer studies are conducted, such studies have to use patients in an open society (roaming free), recalling what they ate, and the patients would have to be observed over time. These types of studies have been done and have been shown to have their own inherent problems and biases. Because such studies have flaws and aren't definitive, the "experts" weigh in with their opinions. And you know the old saying about opinions (expert or not): Everybody's got one.

So, these "expert" opinions get pushed (or not), based on a host of factors that have zero to do with science—political agendas, corporate interests, the expert's popularity, etc. And the result is mass confusion. If a media outlet reports that a "study" says eating X is good for you, people tend to believe it. Why? Well it was a "scientific study," and it was reported in the news, so it must be true, right? Not exactly. Some studies aren't designed well. In fact, some are designed to prove the point of the person doing the study, regardless of what the science reveals. By the time the truth gets out, it is overshadowed by the misinformation, which tends to stick.

That's just how the confusion about the supposed danger of eating fat began in the first place. To untangle that web, let's look back at a researcher named Ancel Keys, a prominent University of Minnesota-based physiologist, who first popularized the idea that consuming too much fat leads to heart disease. Keys' research was so influential that his face was featured on the cover of *Time* magazine on Jan. 13, 1961.

In his book, *Good Calories, Bad Calories: Fats, Carbs, and the Contro-*

versial Science of Diet and Health, Science Writer Gary Taubes presents the case of Keys. Earlier in his career, Keys had worked on starvation studies and during World War II developed the non-perishable, high-calorie pocket meals, known as K-rations, for soldiers. The "K" is widely believed to be short for Keys. He later became interested in heart disease and in 1953 made a presentation that would lead to his so-called "diet-heart hypothesis." During a symposium at Mount Sinai Hospital in New York, Keys presented a graph of historical data from six countries, showing a direct link between death from degenerative heart disease (coronary disease, angina pectoris, infarction, chronic myocarditis, and myocardial degeneration) and fat intake. The graph showed that in those six countries—England and Wales, Australia, Canada, Italy, Japan, and United States—the higher the fat, the higher the degenerative heart disease. Later that year, Keys published a paper on the topic.

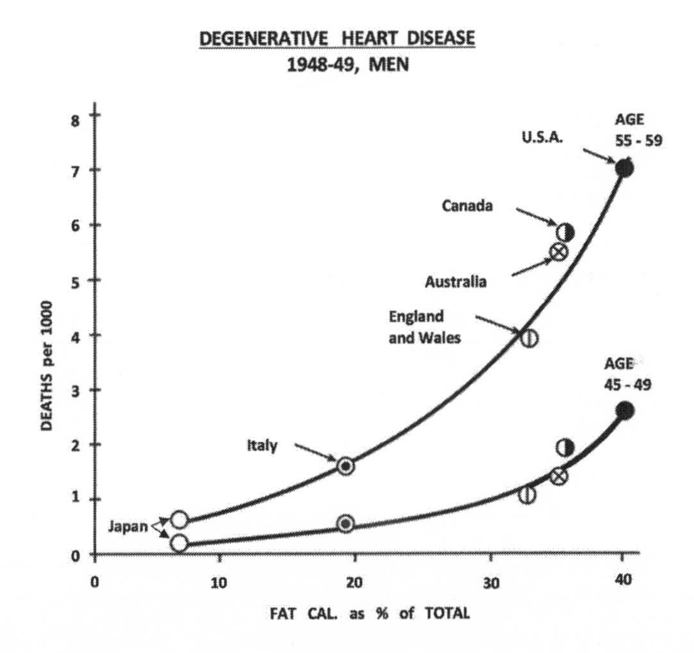

The problem was, Keys presented data from only those six select countries, when data was available for twenty-two countries. When the complete data from all of the countries was tracked, it showed no significant correlation between fat intake and heart disease. Four years later in 1957, two other scientists (Drs. J. Yerushalmy and H.E. Hilleboe) published the complete data and findings for a three-year period from 1951-1953. In their paper they noted that out of the thirteen countries that ate more than 30 percent fat, the majority of those countries had a lower death rate, not a higher one. More specifically, they stated that six countries had deaths rates greater than 400 (per 100,000 people) compared to seven countries that had deaths rates LESS than 400 (per 100,000 people). However, by then, Keys' diet-heart hypothesis was all but doctrine. Since that time, no definitive evidence has shown a correlation between heart disease and fat intake. In fact, a stack of evidence has shown the opposite: that high-carb intake, such as the consumption of sugary beverages, is directly associated with heart disease and stroke. High-carb intake can also lead to pre-diabetes, diabetes, and metabolic syndrome. As a matter of fact, diabetes leads to a two-to-fourfold increase in the rate of cardiovascular disease and a two-to-fourfold (that's 200%-400%) increase risk of death from cardiovascular disease.

Drs. Yerushalmy and Hilleboe: Mortality From Arteriosclerotic and Degenerative Heart Disease and Fat Calories From 22 Countries in Men 55-59 Years Old

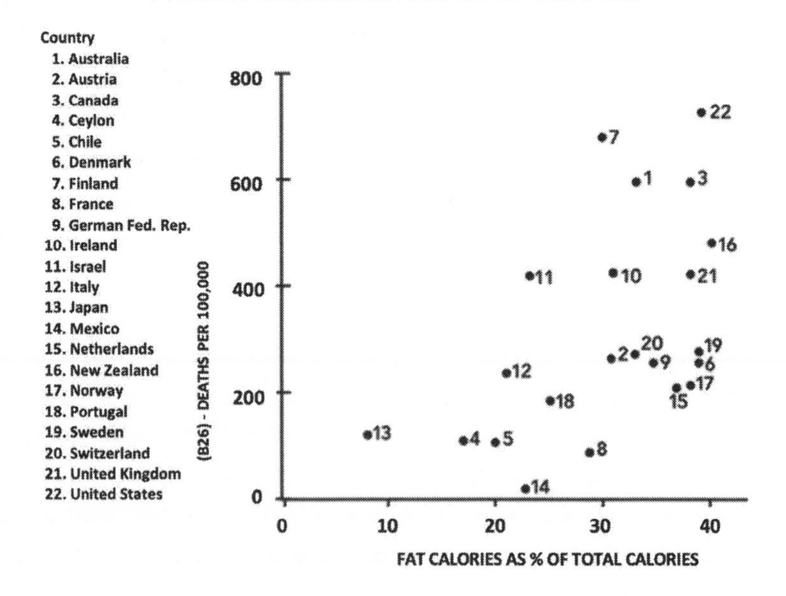

Side-by-side Comparison: Ancel Keys Graph (on left – 6 Countries) and Yerushalmy and Hilleboe (on right – 22 Countries)

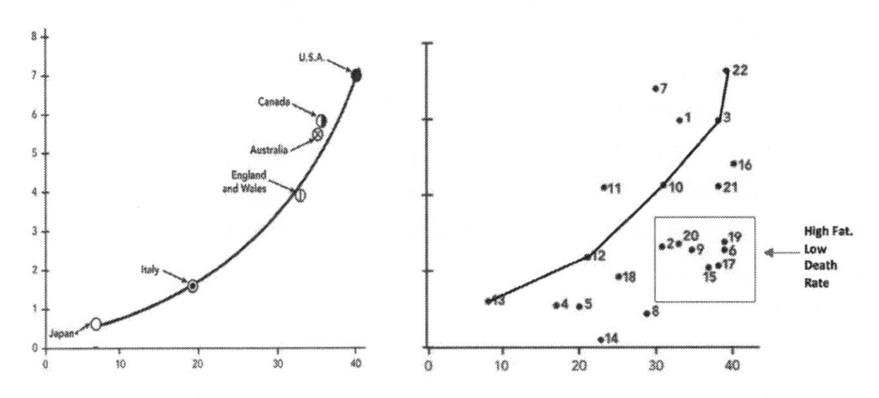

So why did Keys use only six countries instead of the data from all twenty-two countries? I think it was because he wanted to prove what he believed. Nowadays, such scientific data would have been reviewed by the doctor's peers before publication in a scientific journal. But that was not always the case at the time, and as the creator of the K-Rations, Keys was a very popular figure. It has been said that he was also known to be a bit of a bully who pushed his ideas with a fury that aimed to crush those who disagreed with him. He never backed down from his claims about fat and heart disease. In 1958, Keys even embarked on an actual study to prove his theory, since the publication of the data from the six countries was not an actual study. This time, he chose seven countries, and again, he chose seven that he knew would favor his conclusion, omitting countries that he thought may not prove his hypothesis.

With the deck stacked in favor of Keys' diet-heart hypothesis, his seven-country study, which he first wrote about in a 1980 book published by Harvard University Press (but even earlier in the journal *Acta Medica Scandinavica* in 1967), showed that saturated fats had a linear relationship to degenerative heart disease. The new graph wasn't quite as impressive as the cherry-picked data from the initial six countries, though. The seven-country study showed a correlation only between saturated fat (not total fat) and heart disease. Thus, Keys adjusted his fat theory and focused only on saturated fat. It didn't matter that other studies showed that people in other countries consumed high levels of saturated fats and experienced very low rates of heart disease—people like the Maasai in Africa. Keys dismissed this data, as he had earlier. His seven-country study solidified the diet-heart hypothesis. He had enough influence to stifle his detractors, and they all but withered away.

Low-fat Hype

As Keys persuaded the country that saturated fat in the diet was bad for coronary health, in stepped Senator George McGovern. The Democratic senator from South Dakota had been charged by the White House to come up with dietary guidelines for Americans. Sweden already had developed guidelines, and America wanted to lead the way in recommending to its citizens what to eat for better health, especially heart health. Studies had begun to show that heart disease was on the rise in the United States.

Before his committee was commissioned, Senator McGovern was at a month-long retreat hosted by multi-millionaire Nathan Pritikin, then a prominent, self-proclaimed diet expert. Pritikin wasn't a physician, but he commissioned other physicians to conduct studies that he often funded (possibly resulting in bias). Pritikin preached a low-fat, high-carb diet. He proclaimed he had cured diabetes and helped many patients get off their diabetes medicines by feeding them a low-fat, high-carb diet (I heard him say this on a television interview he did for PBS). Given what we know today about diabetes, that isn't logical and likely was not true. Feeding a diabetic a significant amount of sugar or refined carbohydrates would raise the patient's blood sugar levels, requiring more medicines, not less. And a high-carb, low-fat diet likely wouldn't cure anyone's diabetes. McGovern and his wife didn't stay for the whole retreat, but they were convinced of Pritikin's teachings about the benefits of a low-fat diet for heart health. Senator McGovern later assigned one of his employees to write the dietary guidelines. The aide who was given that task had no scientific background or expertise; he consulted with another low-fat proponent who was a Harvard professor and nutritionist. The aide ended up writing the dietary guidelines for all Americans, forming the basis of the federal recommendations that still recommend and focus on fat reduction.

Investigative journalist Nina Teicholz also writes about Keys' influence on the low-fat movement in her 2014 book, *The Big Fat Surprise: Why Butter, Meat, and Cheese Belong in a Healthy Diet.* In it, she makes the case for how quickly the media also got on the bandwagon, spreading the low-fat hype. According to Teicholz and Taubes, the powers that be didn't feel they had the time to wait another decade or more to get more definitive information on the low-fat diet before recommending it to an entire population. Corporate America fell in line, developing an array of low-fat (and by definition, high-carb) foods. By the late 1970s, researchers believed a low-fat diet would be the answer to addressing not just heart disease, but also obesity. At the time, about 12 percent of Americans had obesity. Low-fat advocates estimated that obesity and heart disease would go away by the turn of the century (the year 2000). They were dead wrong, literally.

Americans wholeheartedly bought into the low-fat diet craze, and our consumption of fat dropped from about 40-plus percent to the recommended 30 percent or less from the 1970s to 2015. But as we all know, the obesity rate didn't go down. In fact, it grew at an alarming rate. Somehow, following those low-fat guidelines must have made Americans hungrier because we ultimately ate more, not less, consuming a low-fat, high-carbohydrate diet that increased our calorie intake at least 10 percent from the 1970s to today, according to the federal Centers for Disease Control and Prevention and United States Department of Agriculture (USDA). Some studies show the percentage of calories increased even higher, by about 20 percent. At any rate, obesity has more than tripled since the 1970s, and the rate of heart disease has skyrocketed. Fortunately, deaths from the increase in heart disease have not increased as dramatically, which is likely a result of the cholesterol-lowering statin drugs, as well as stents and coronary artery bypass surgery. Americans have eaten less fat since the 1970s, but we've become fatter, according to the CDC's National Health and Nutrition Examination Survey. Why?

Some might argue that it's not the low-fat craze that caused the obesity epidemic, but excess calories and lack of exercise. The average calorie intake in the 1970s was 2,025 calories, versus 2,481 in 2010, a 23 percent increase. That sounds convincing, but for the last almost two decades,

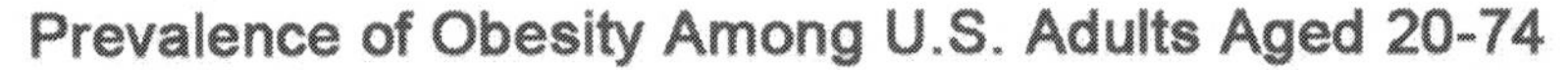

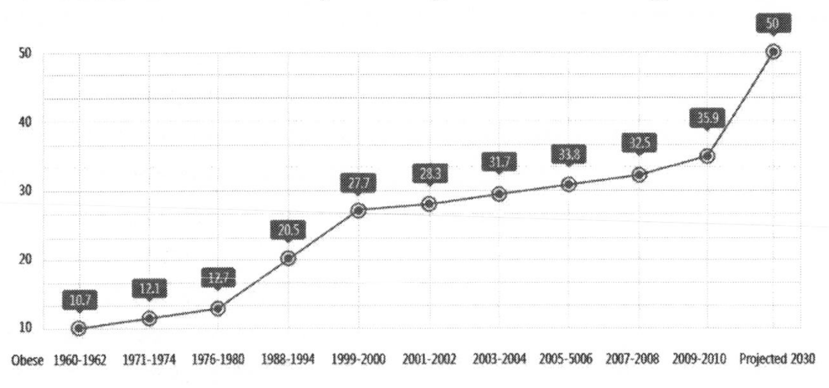

Derived from NHANES data (http://www.cdc.gov/nchs/data/hestat/obesity_adult_09_10/obesity_adult_09_10.html#table1)

Americans' intake of calories has been about the same, yet obesity has continued to grow steadily, about 1 percent to 2 percent every year. So if we are eating roughly the same amount of calories, why are we still gaining weight? Well, following the calories in-calories out logic, if we are not eating more, then we must be more physically inactive. So, let's look at that. Data from an analysis of that topic (from stateofobesity.org) shows that we are no less physically inactive today than we were ten years ago. In fact, our physical inactivity has stayed about the same over the last decade. Plus, gym memberships continue to rise year after year, so some might say we are more active than a decade ago.

U.S health club membership over a 20-year period

22.00%
20.00%
18.00%
16.00%
14.00%
12.00%
10.00%
1995 1997 1999 2001 2003 2005 2007 2009 2011 2013 2015

Granted, just because people have a gym membership doesn't mean they actually are going to the gym. But at the very least we can say we are no more inactive today than we were a decade ago, especially if we take into account the various physical activity marketing campaigns, such as First Lady Michelle Obama's "Let's Move" campaign. Yet, obesity continues to rise.

So if we are not consuming more calories and our physical activity is roughly the same (or maybe even slightly increased), why are we still gaining weight at such alarming rates? To answer that question, we have to throw out the old logic. Calories in do not equal calories out. It is the type of calories we eat (excessive sugars and refined carbohydrates) that determines where the energy goes—whether it is burned or stored (something called fuel partitioning, which we will talk about later). Sugars and refined carbohydrates dictate that process through insulin production, regardless of calories. The 250 calories from a kale salad is not the same as the 250 calories from a Snickers bar. The increase in obesity likely has to do with increasing insulin resistance. The longer the body is exposed to constant high levels of carbs, the more insulin resistant the body becomes, and thus more obesity develops.

Another point about the calories in-calories out theory: Physical activity (which includes exercise and other non-structured movement that burns calories) plays a smaller role in losing weight than some may realize; it accounts for just about 20 percent of weight loss. The other 80 percent is diet. Don't get me wrong, I recommend getting the benefit of that 20 percent from physical activity (besides, physical activity places a bigger role in overall heart health and other medical issues, so it is very important), but *the* most significant factor in weight loss is diet, and that is where the main focus should be, particularly in the beginning. My program gets participants to start losing weight by first focusing on changing their diet and then on safely building physical activity into their regular routine, so that they won't get hurt.

There's one more study that makes the case that Americans may have been too quick to demonize dietary saturated fats and that the truth was purposely hidden: the Minnesota Coronary Experiment. Between 1968 and 1973, researchers who were associates of Ancel Keys (who was also an author on the paper) conducted the tightly-controlled experiment, which involved more than 9,000 patients. It was a huge study in terms of nutritional research, one of the largest (if not *the* largest) nutritional study ever done under the best research parameters. This study (as unethical as it was) was done the way an ideal study of nutrition would need to be conducted. The researchers used institutionalized patients (living in six state mental hospitals and one nursing home), and the patients were able to eat only what the researchers fed them. Then they were monitored to see what would happen to them. Because of how unethical it was, a study like this could never be done today. Nonetheless, this would be considered a definitive study. The investigators conducting the study were stunned when results showed that people who ate a diet rich in saturated fats did *not* have more heart disease than those who ate a diet rich in polyunsaturated fat from vegetable oil. The study went unpublished for sixteen years.

The researchers finally revealed some of the results in 1989 in a medical journal that didn't attract many readers. When asked why the findings were kept silent for so long, one of the lead scientists involved in the study stated, "We were just so disappointed in the way they turned out." The researchers didn't like the results, so they kept them quiet, even as the public continued to believe that eating a diet high in saturated fats would cause heart disease. Even more compelling, after the lead investigator had died and the rest of the data that they had concealed was turned over by the lead investigator's son and analyzed, it showed that while those in the low-saturated fat group experienced just a modest decrease in cholesterol (30 points), they had a 22 percent increased risk of death. It's hard to say whether the low-fat diet was the sole cause of the deaths.

It is not unusual for studies to show conflicting results. How does science rectify that? A method called a *meta-analysis* is one remedy. Basically, all of the relevant studies are combined and analyzed to determine if the preponderance of evidence is for or against the proposed question. Remember when the news reported coffee was bad for your health? Those media reports were based on a 1973 study in the *New England Journal of Medicine* of more than 12,000 patients. The study found that drinking one to five cups of coffee a day increased the risk of heart attacks by 60 percent. The study also showed that drinking six or more cups a day doubled that risk to 120 percent. Another study reported in 1978 in the *New England Journal of Medicine* found a short-term rise in blood pressure after three cups of coffee. Authors called for further research into caffeine and hypertension. A decade after the initial coffee study, *The British Medical Journal* reported that people who drank coffee were 17 percent less likely to die early during the study period from any cause, 19 percent less likely to die of heart disease, and 18 percent less likely to develop cancer, compared to people who did not drink coffee. Which is correct? Based on a review of meta-analyses of that question, published in 2017, coffee is good for you, at least in moderation (ahhhh, I love my coffee).

A meta-analysis also was conducted to answer the question: "Does saturated fat cause cardiovascular disease?" The analysis showed that saturated fat neither causes heart attacks nor helps to prevent them. A number of meta-analysis studies have shown the same repeatedly. One large (approximately 340,000 patients) meta-analysis, published by *The British Medical Journal* in 2015, showed the same. So once and for all, dietary fats, in particular saturated fats, do not increase your risk of heart attack or stroke.

Got it?

Good.

In a nutshell, going on a low-fat diet to prevent heart disease and obesity is a fifty-year experiment that failed, and we are fatter and sicker because of it, primarily because we substituted the fat with sugars and refined carbohydrates, which are more deadly. Americans have more obesity than we've ever had before, and we continue to grow, outpacing even the experts' estimates. Did you know that even though Americans have decreased their fat intake by 10 percent (from 40 percent to 30 percent), obesity has risen by almost 300 percent? So much for curing obesity with a low-fat diet by the year 2000. Plus, as a result of obesity, Americans also are the sickest we have ever been. In medicine, we classify the disease of obesity into two categories: (1) fat mass disease and (2) sick fat disease (adiposopathy). The "fat mass disease" category is made up of the diseases caused or worsened just by the sheer excess weight, including sleep apnea, which shuts off your airway (suffocates you) when you sleep, asthma, and arthritis (particularly in weight bearing joints, like the knee). The second category, "sick fat disease," or adiposopathy, is the disease of the fat cell itself. The fat cell is a bad player once it becomes "sick," which leads to a host of other diseases and increased risk of blood clots and cancers.

There are a number of other health conditions associated with obesity, including stroke, hypertension, cataracts, pulmonary issues, and more.

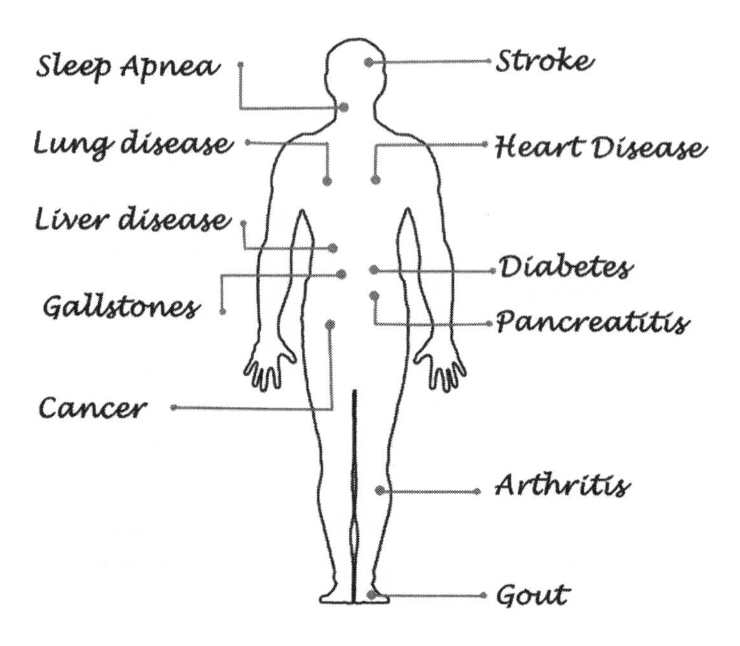

We can't afford to go another ten or twenty years with the same diet dogma. It's time to change course. Let's start with making the case that in general, fat does not make you fat. There is some evidence that polyunsaturated fats, like vegetable oils, can increase your risk of death, (namely by increasing your hemorrhagic stroke and cancer risk). *Dietary* fat on the whole, however (specifically saturated fat), not only does not increase your risk of heart disease, it also does not make you fat, despite what you've heard. The real culprits are sugar and refined carbohydrates. Even though fat has more calories per gram than sugar (nine calories per gram for fat, versus four calories per gram for sugar and protein), sugar still makes you fatter than fat. I don't normally use the word "fat" to describe obesity, as it's considered a derogatory term. My intent is simply to debunk the "fat makes you fat" myth. The fat we eat isn't the same as the fat that's made in our bodies. Dietary fat does not automatically turn into body fat. To understand what really makes us gain weight, we have to understand insulin (a growth and fat storage hormone) and how it works. A low-carb diet that is high in fat and protein does not significantly stimulate insulin production. If you don't produce much insulin, you won't store much fat; in fact, your body will burn fat. And what makes your body produce a significant amount of insulin? Drum roll, please ... carbohydrates.

If we consider malnourishment among children in Third World countries, it reveals much about how carbs are metabolized. Kwashiorkor is a kind of malnutrition that results from a diet that has the appropriate caloric intake but is nutritionally poor because it is based primarily on carbs (sugars and refined carbs) with a severe lack of protein. Children with kwashiorkor experience a change in their physical appearance after they are weaned from their mother's protein-rich breast milk, 25 percent of which is saturated fat. Your brain is also 60 percent fat—25 percent of all the cholesterol in your body is contained in your brain, which is only 2 percent of your body weight. So cholesterol is important for the brain. When they begin eating a diet that consists primarily of sugar and refined carbohydrates, such as bread, rice, etc., they begin to develop bloated bellies and fatty livers while their arms and legs become very skinny, with no muscle mass. They have significant fat in their bellies and livers. How can this be if they are starving? The consumption of high levels of carbs raises their level of insulin, which drives the carbs into storage as fat and breaks down whatever muscle is present as energy instead. That's how powerful insulin is.

On the other end of the spectrum is another type of malnutrition, called marasmus, which happens when there is an equal deficiency of all food and the body just wastes away.

However, in other cultures, such as the Maasai tribe in Africa, where

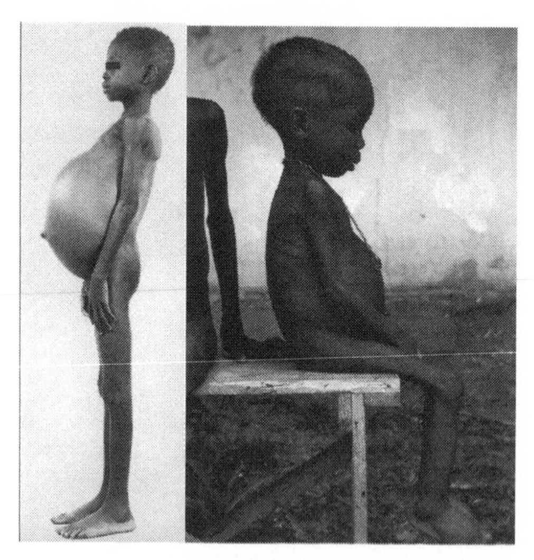

Kwashiorkor

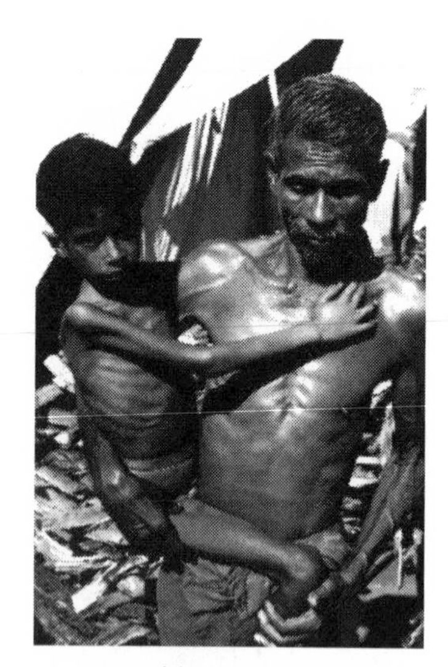

Marasmus

the diet is rich in protein and fat with virtually no carbs (i.e. a low-carb diet), the people grow tall, lean, muscular and have prowess. Carbs are not an essential nutrient. The reason humans don't need carbs (like we need certain proteins and fats) is because our bodies can make carbs through a process called gluconeogenesis. You can be healthy without eating carbs at all, as evidenced by the Maasai and other cultures, such as the Inuit and Native Americans (before they were westernized).

People suffering from kwashiorkor are similar to those Americans who

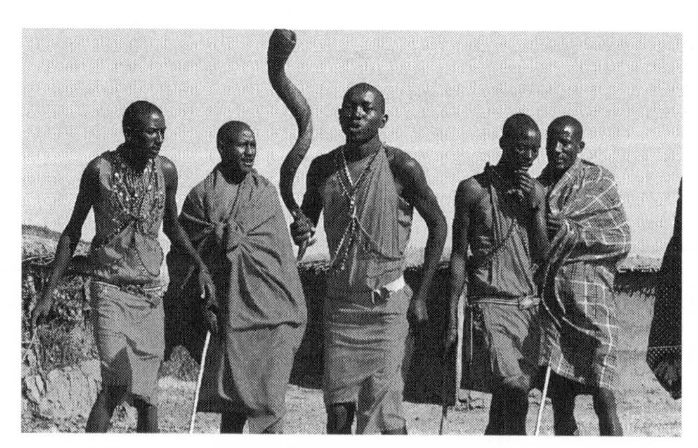

Maasai

overdo it with beer and develop a "beer belly." Beer is mostly a sugar called maltose, and it, too, triggers an insulin response that is very similar to what happens with kwashiorkor.

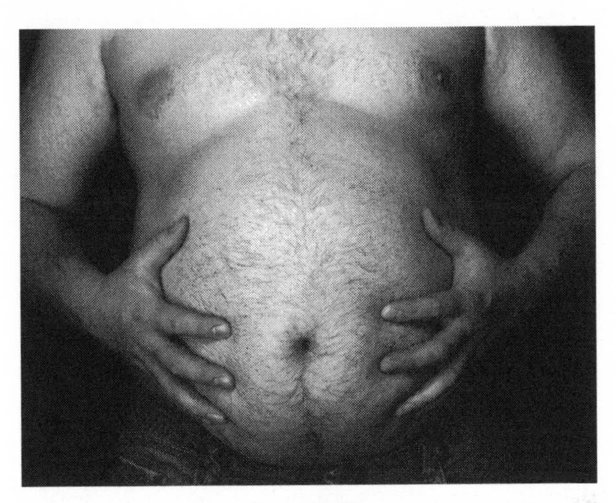

Beer Belly

So, what happens when we eat fat? Some of the fat we eat is not absorbed and goes out in our stool. The fat that is absorbed gets broken down in your intestines by pancreatic enzymes and bile acid. The broken-down fat is transported across the intestinal membrane into your bloodstream as triglycerides (of note, carbohydrates are also turned into triglycerides in your liver). The triglycerides are used as energy by muscle cells, and some are stored locally in the muscle cell, where they can be used for energy at a later time. Thus, most of the *fat* you eat is used as energy and whatever's leftover can be stored as fat. This reminds me of another point to debunk the "calories in equals calories out" myth. If every calorie you eat is absorbed (meaning everything you eat is broken down and taken into your bloodstream), then by definition nothing should come out of your body because all of the calories are absorbed. Thus, that means none of us should ever have stool.

With a low-carb diet, your body produces low insulin levels, which allows the flow of energy out of fat cells, resulting in weight loss. This is very similar to what fasting or intermittent fasting does. Your insulin is low when you fast (since there are no carbohydrates, as well as no fat, or protein) and you burn fat. (So these diets operate basically like a low-carb diet). When higher levels of insulin are produced with a high-carb diet, the flow of energy is into fat cells, resulting in weight gain. In other words, if you eat a low-fat/high-carb diet (with 60 percent or more of your food from carbs), the carbs are used as the energy source, not allowing you to burn fat. The rest of the carbs are eventually stored as fat, which can lead to obesity. This increase in fat also can lead to insulin resistance, which means the cells throughout your body have difficulty absorbing the glucose, and sugar builds up in your bloodstream, which triggers even more fat storage. (When your body becomes insulin resistant it goes in this order: first the muscles become resistant, then the liver and last, fat. So when your other cells are becoming resistant, your fat cells are saying, "Bring it on, I'll take all the excess!") It's a vicious cycle. You eat carbs, which make you hungry after a few hours, and so you eat more carbs. And then you just produce more fat. To maintain a normal healthy blood sugar level, there should be no more than the equivalent of about a teaspoon of sugar circulating throughout your entire body at any given time. (We eat more than a teaspoon, or 4 grams, of sugar every day, but our body uses much of that as energy and stores the rest.)

If your sugar is really high, your body tries to get rid of it through your urine (Before blood tests, that's how we knew you were diabetic. A doctor actually would taste your urine to see if it tasted sweet.) If that doesn't work—i.e., your body can no longer regulate your sugar level—it goes too high in your blood and you become diabetic.

I don't want to vilify carbohydrates as a whole the way fat has been vilified for the past fifty years. As a matter of fact, my No Guesswork Plan gradually allows you to add some healthy carbs, such as whole grains and fiber (fiber is a component of whole grains), back into your diet in the maintenance phase. It's a blended low-carb Mediterranean diet. (A Mediterranean diet has been shown to be the best for the heart.) You will learn more about that phase when I describe the plan later in the book.

So why is a low-fat diet still being promoted in certain sectors as the healthiest option? Why not tell the public the truth about fat, and thus, the truth about sugar and refined carbs? My speculation is that some powerful people in powerful positions really believe their point of view—that a low-fat diet is healthier. And dare I say there may be financial incentives to keeping things the way they are (at the expense of American lives). Because there are so many factors that play into why people develop and are unable to reverse obesity, it is easy to consider only the factors that fit your point of view. And so for the last 50 years, low-fat advocates have tried to explain away the data that clearly shows that fats aren't bad for your health. Or, they ignore the data altogether. As I mentioned, we would have to lock people in an experimental society for decades and study them to get absolute data. So the confusion continues, and which side you choose is almost like a religion. But what can't be refuted is the belief fifty years ago that a low-fat diet would cure heart disease and obesity. That never happened; in fact, the opposite is true. A low-fat diet (and thus, a high carb diet) coincides with increases in obesity, diabetes, cancer (even when you take out the statistics from lung cancer caused by smoking), Alzheimer's, heart disease, and stroke.

Given the state of the nation's health, the current generation of children is predicted to die sooner than the generation before them. That should give us pause. For the sake of our children and the next generation, let's at least consider eating and living another way.

CHAPTER THREE

The Hunger Gremlin

Let's talk about the system that controls your hunger and cravings. It's all about the body's set point—the state your body perceives as normal. The human body has a number of set points—a set point for your temperature (98.6 F), your pH (7.40), and your weight (or better stated, your fat mass). Your body is really good at maintaining all of its set points. The set point theory on weight holds that, based on genetics (and a host of other factors that can change your set point such as stress, menopause, environment, etc.), each of us has a weight range that is considered normal to our bodies. That range varies from person to person. When your body perceives a threat to what it considers normal, such as significant weight loss, certain defense mechanisms kick in to try to return your body to its set point.

Your body can't make you grab a Big Mac, but it can change your hormones and neurotransmitters to make you feel hunger and cravings, and it can suppress the hormones and neurotransmitters that make you feel satiated (satisfied). Under those circumstances, you are likely to go out and seek whatever you crave. So, it's no wonder that it's sometimes tough to lose weight and even tougher to keep it off. The majority of people who lose weight (upwards of 80 percent) gain it right back. But knowing why and how it happens gives us the tools we need to overcome the body's tendencies.

The hormone responsible for causing cravings and hunger is called ghrelin. It's one of the "gut hormones," and it's produced primarily in your stomach. I call ghrelin "the Hunger Gremlin."

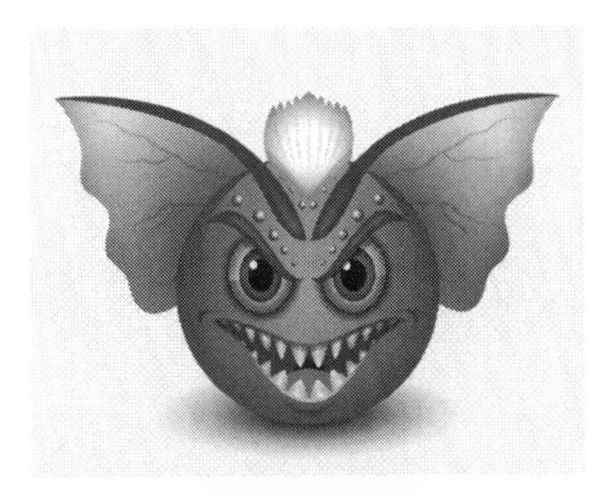

Here's how it works:

Ghrelin is low just after a meal. As you get closer to your next meal, ghrelin starts to increase, making you feel hungry. Your level of ghrelin continues to rise—and so does your level of hunger—the closer it gets to mealtime. Moments before you eat, ghrelin is at its peak. Afterwards, your ghrelin level and your appetite plummet, and the cycle starts all over again. Think of it this way: When you eat, the Hunger Gremlin shrinks, but as mealtime approaches, the little monster grows, making you feel more and more ravenous until the beast is fed.

Ghrelin activates your craving center, which is known as the limbic system. This system is mainly located in four parts of your brain: the hypothalamus, thalamus, amygdala, and hippocampus. When your craving center is activated, the other area of your brain responsible for helping you to reason (the pre-frontal cortex), is blocked. Thus, there is no way to get a message to your craving center to manage the actual craving. It's as if the craving center is spinning so fast that your reasoning center can't get inside to interact; the craving center just spins and spins and spins.

There are just two known ways to stop your craving center from spinning. One is to wait for about twenty minutes or so, and the spinning naturally slows down. At that time, your reasoning center can then interact, and usually the craving decreases. This strategy is often used to help people with drug addiction manage cravings. People with drug addiction in treatment are often counseled that if a craving occurs, they have to fight it for just twenty minutes before the spinning slows enough for them to make a rational decision to say no. Likewise, when a food craving seems unbearable, if you can fight it for twenty minutes, the strong desire for a certain food will decrease on its own.

Ghrelin also activates hunger/appetite. This happens through an area of your brain called the arcuate nucleus, your appetite center, which is your appetite/hunger hub. So, not only does ghrelin ignite cravings, but by activating your appetite center, that sneaky gremlin also makes you hungry. Given those facts, it's easy to see how difficult it can be to resist tempting foods!

The second way to stop the craving center from spinning works like this: Say you see some freshly cooked, crispy fries, salted just the way you like them, with that addictive smell drawing you closer to them. Of course, by now your craving center is spinning out of control. You know you're not supposed to eat them, but you can't reason because your craving center is lit up and spinning at top speed. And the area of your brain responsible for reasoning can't get inside. So, what do you do? You eat the fries, and your craving center immediately stops spinning (since you satisfied the craving). By the time your reasoning center comes in, it's already too late. You've eaten the fries, and now you feel guilty. Fortunately, those are not the only two options. Another strategy I share with my patients is to stop their craving center from spinning in the first place. The way to do that is to decrease the ghrelin in your body so that it doesn't activate your cravings. And what decreases ghrelin? Protein.

If we can decrease ghrelin, we can decrease hunger and cravings and have better control of what we eat and how much of it we eat. Of all the three macronutrients—fat, carbohydrates, and protein—protein has the biggest effect on ghrelin. So, a strategy we use in our clinic to help patients avoid getting hungry is to instruct them to eat protein between meals. Feed the beast and keep it satisfied. That way, the patients won't feel ravenous when they sit down to eat their next meal, and they likely will have better control. But even if patients are not hungry when they sit down for their next meal, I urge them to eat something (preferably protein and healthy fats) to keep their ghrelin level as low as possible. With a low ghrelin level, patients are able to make more rational decisions about what and how much they eat. I also encourage my patients to eat plenty of healthy fats to add variety and satisfaction to their meals. I will explain later on what I mean by healthy fats (it includes more than what you may think).

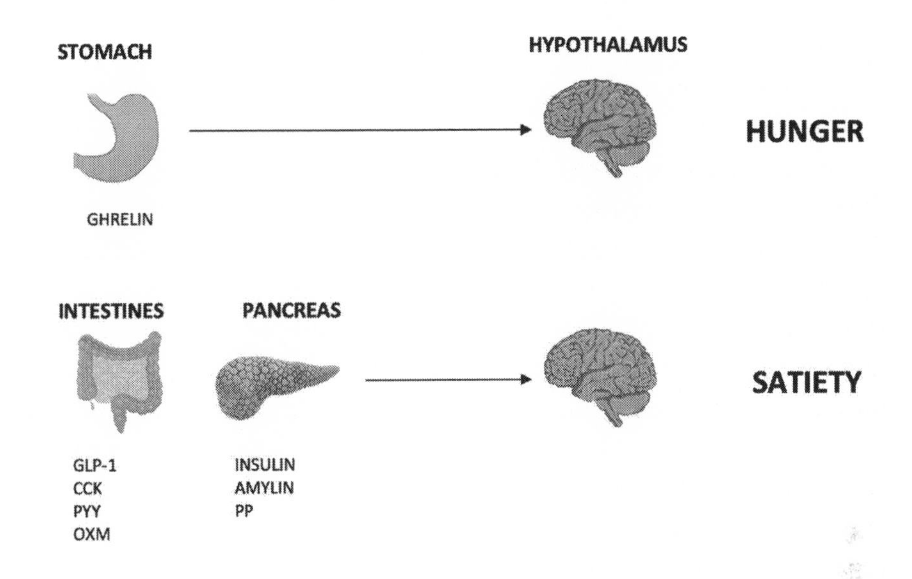

Let's talk more about your craving center, called the limbic system. It's a powerful driver of cravings through the secretion of dopamine, a chemical that acts as a kind of messenger between brain cells. These messengers are called neurotransmitters. Sugar and refined carbohydrates light up the limbic system more than any other type of food. In fact, if you take a functional MRI of the area of the brain where the limbic system resides, carbs light it up even more than cocaine (see image on www.noguesswork.com). That means a craving for carbs is even more powerful than the craving for drugs. That is in part what I mean when I tell patients on their first visit with me in the clinic that obesity is not their fault and that their body is working against them.

In addition to causing obesity, eating sugars and refined carbohydrates in large amounts (in excess of 150 grams per day) causes the body to crave even more carbs. This sets up a vicious cycle that is difficult to break. Fats also can light up the craving center, but to a lesser degree than carbs. And as I mentioned, protein *slows down* the limbic system. I repeat: eating protein decreases ghrelin. So, a diet that is low in carbs (particularly low in sugars and refined carbohydrates) and higher in fats and protein constitutes a well-formulated low-carb diet. This kind of meal plan enables you to control your diet, instead of your diet controlling you.

Size Doesn't Matter! (at least not in bariatric surgery)

To better understand the role of ghrelin (the Hunger Gremlin) in sabotaging weight loss, look no further than bariatric procedures, which are used often as a last resort to help patients with obesity lose weight. It was long believed that bariatric surgery works because it shrinks the stomach, so patients get full quicker. But researchers later learned that there was another—perhaps more significant—reason. Of the three main types of bariatric surgery, the most effective is the gastric bypass (technically called Roux-en-Y). The gastric bypass cuts out about 80 percent of the stomach and then moves the intestines closer to the stomach. This process dramatically reduces the size of the stomach, which also results in a reduction of about 80 percent of the patient's ghrelin. Also, moving the intestine closer to the stomach triggers the release of intestinal hormones that make the patient feel satisfied quicker.

The next most successful procedure is called a "sleeve," which also reduces the stomach by 80 percent and shrinks the Hunger Gremlin by the same percentage. The least effective procedure is the Lap Band, which puts a band around the stomach to make it smaller but doesn't remove ghrelin from the stomach or aid in releasing the other hormones in the intestine to make the patient satisfied. As a result, many of people who get the Lap Band either don't lose a significant amount of weight or regain the weight within two years.

What does this tell us about the Hunger Gremlin? It is such a powerful, irresistible force that even when the stomach is physically smaller, most patients cannot resist the urge to eat.

TYPES OF BARIATRIC SURGERY

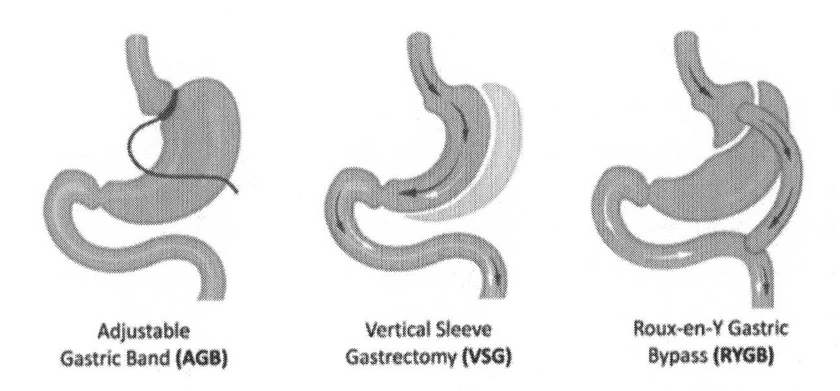

This explains why we get hungry and crave food. The ability to resist is not just about willpower. Sure, you can try to will your way through the sensation of hunger and cravings for a little while, but there is a real metabolic reason why you feel so hungry and a real reason that this battle isn't easy to win.

Willpower

Of course, you're probably wondering about the role of willpower. Most of the time when I say obesity is not a matter of willpower, I get a funny look from the person I'm talking to. Even after I explain the science, the needle moves only a bit, and they still don't completely buy it. Willpower is a tricky concept. Let me explain. Sure, you can use willpower to get through things for a couple days, a couple of weeks, or a couple of months, even; but few people can use willpower this way day after day, year after year. I can think of only a handful of people, like Ghandi, who were successful at it for years. And I would venture to say that most of us don't have Ghandi's willpower.

The bottom line is, it's not a good strategy to use willpower as your *primary* means of getting to a healthier weight. That is a losing strategy. Your body will fight you for years to return to your baseline weight. It's better to understand what the body is doing to defend what it perceives as normal, and use that information to devise a strategy to reach a healthy weight. Why not use the right tool for the job? Sure, use willpower, if it can help you shed the weight. But there's a better strategy. I suggest you use your willpower to work on the NGW plan.

The one qualifier I will mention here is… TRACKING AND PLANNING. This does have something to do with willpower. Your body is not making you *NOT* track or *NOT* plan, that's all you. So, this is the one area where I will admit that discipline and willpower play a very significant role in your success to get to a healthier weight.

Gut Hormones

As I mentioned previously, the hormone ghrelin (the Hunger Gremlin) activates your hunger and craving centers. This is counterbalanced by a number of other hormones in your gut that help to keep you satisfied. All of this is regulated in your brain, and the thermostat in your brain is responsible for regulating your body weight. Wherever that thermostat is set, your body does everything it can to keep your "temperature" at that set "weight." So when you attempt to lose weight, your body jumps into action to get you back to what it perceives as normal, releasing ghrelin in your stomach, which sets off your cravings and makes you hungry. At the same time, the hormones in your gut that counteract ghrelin—GLP-1, OXM, PP, CCK, leptin, insulin, and amylin—are effectively suppressed.

Ghrelin and Other Gut Hormones That Help Regulate Your Thermostat (i.e. Set Point)

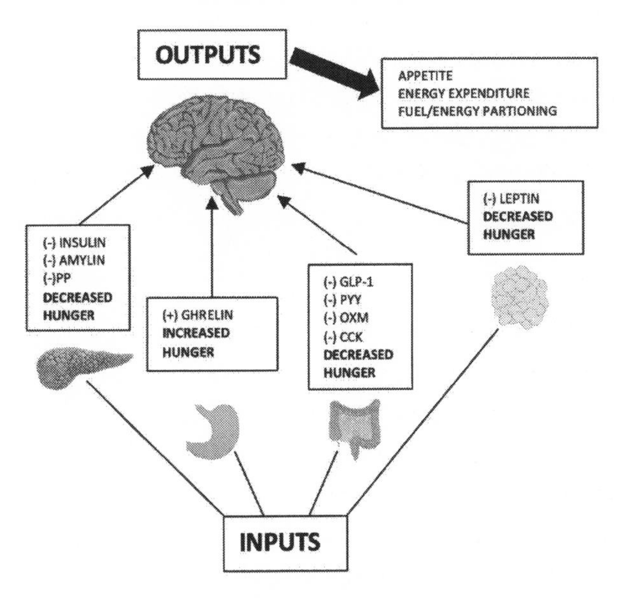

This picture is a basic schematic of how your body controls your brain to regulate your body weight. I break it down into two parts, your gut hormones and the fat cell signalers (adipokines) and then your metabolism.

You don't have to remember any of these scientific names (and there are a few more I didn't mention), but just know your body has mechanisms to fight cravings and hunger. In fact, studies have been done where a catheter is stuck in the heads of mice and infused with ghrelin, and the mice eat the feed, eat the feed, eat the feed, until they vomit. (Okay rodents don't vomit, but you get the point. They excessively overeat.)

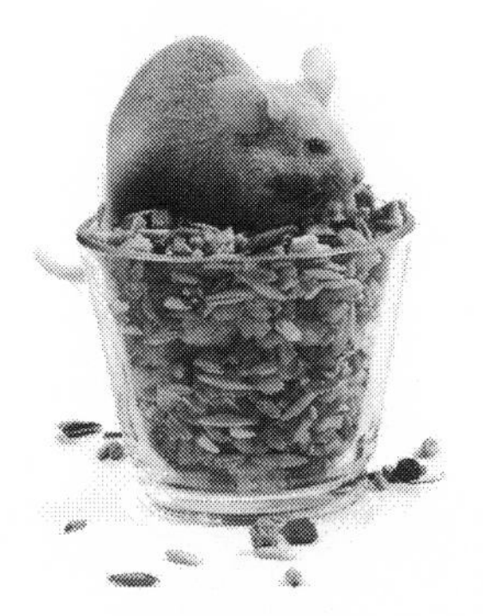

In a second experiment, each mouse's ghrelin supply is blocked, and the mice stare at the feed, stare at the feed, stare at the feed, until they almost starve to death.

Now we can't put catheters in everybody's brain (I wish we could), but if we could, we could cure obesity. Actually, what would be even better is if we knew how to reach into the human brain and change the temperature on that thermostat. In that case, your body would cure obesity for you. We are not there yet, but we are working on it.

Your body is patient; you might think you have willpower, but your body will wait until you are sleep-deprived or have some sort of stress in your life — maybe a bad breakup, financial stress, family problems, etc. When that happens, your body kicks into gear by releasing ghrelin, making you more hungry and intensifying your craving. You won't be able to fight back because the hormones that make you feel satisfied are effectively at ZERO, as your body purposely won't produce them or purposely resists its effects. All the while you're thinking this is happening because you lack willpower, when the truth is your body is working overtime to get you back to your set point.

Leptin

Believe it or not, your fat cells produce signals via hormones that prevent weight gain. One of the more well-known hormones is leptin. Leptin, which decreases appetite and increases your metabolism (energy expenditure), was discovered in 1994 by Jeffrey Friedman and his colleagues. It turned out that mice with a leptin deficiency had obesity, and when you replaced the leptin, the mice lost weight. This was thought to be the obesity Holy Grail. There was so much excitement — the obesity code had finally been cracked! But when researchers gave it to humans, it didn't work. What was the problem? Turns out, obesity made humans leptin resistant (sound familiar?). Just like people with obesity are insulin resistant, they are also leptin resistant. So no matter how much leptin you gave them, it wouldn't work; they didn't lose weight. Scientists discovered that leptin only works in people who are truly leptin deficient. There is a rare genetic disorder where people are leptin deficient, which makes them have obesity.

For these patients, leptin cures obesity. Unfortunately, only a handful of people can benefit from leptin.

Young boy with leptin deficiency (on left) and then after treatment (on right)

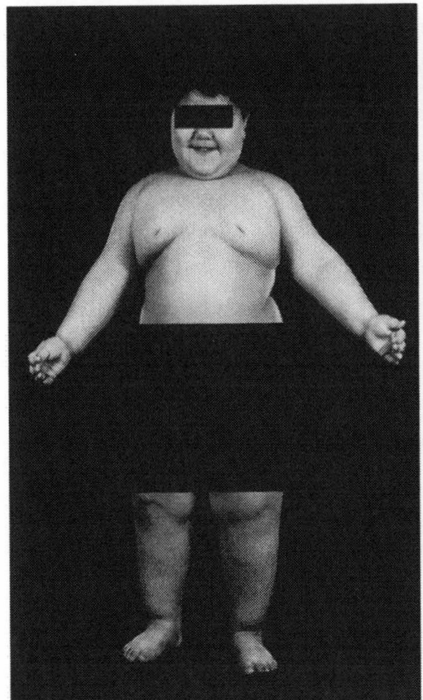

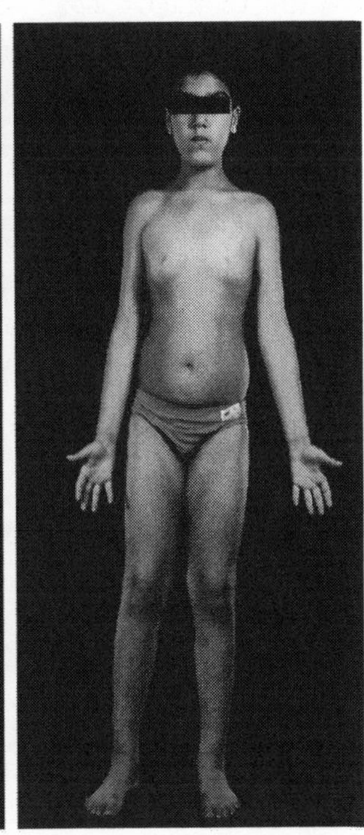

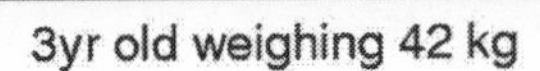

3yr old weighing 42 kg

7yr old weighing 32 kg

So all the hype about leptin was a bust; researchers had to go back to the drawing board. Knowing the mechanisms of how obesity works is helpful, however, in the efforts to find a cure. For example, if we can figure out a way to overcome leptin resistance and activate the leptin receptors to decrease appetite and increase metabolism, science can use that to help people get to a healthier weight. And keep in mind, if you've developed leptin resistance, shedding weight may help you break your resistance naturally so that leptin can do its job and help you better regulate your appetite and metabolism.

Another important signaler that the fat cell produces is adiponectin, which indirectly prevents weight gain by reducing insulin resistance. It also reduces atherosclerosis (blockage of your heart). Unfortunately, in addition to producing leptin and adiponectin, the fat cell also produces a lot of bad stuff, which is why we need to get rid of it. It produces and causes other cells to produce things that cause inflammation, thrombosis, insulin resistance, type 2 diabetes, hypertension, and high cholesterol, among other things. That's why it's so important to get rid of the fat cell and get to a healthier weight.

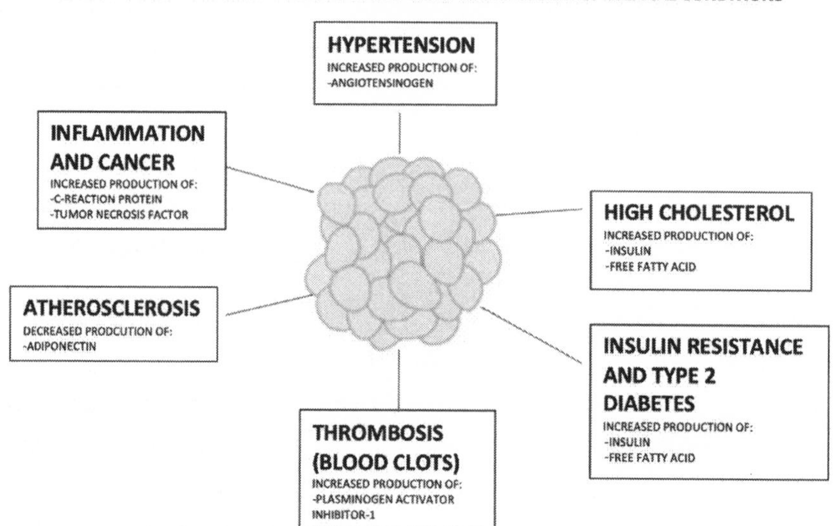

Don't Go Hungry

One of the core strategies of my No Guesswork Plan is to keep the patient satisfied and to keep the Hunger Gremlin at bay. Under my plan, when patients feel the first signs of hunger, I tell them to eat, but just make sure they choose protein or fat. It's that simple. You're not counting calories, so you don't find yourself feeling hungry at 6 p.m. but unable to eat anything because you've reached your caloric intake for the day. If you don't eat, what do you think happens inside to the Hunger Gremlin?

Exactly.

It grows and—more likely than not—wins the battle over willpower.

In fact, that's why I tell my patients to eat on a schedule; that way, they will have something in their stomach well before they feel the first sign of hunger. The Hunger Gremlin will never get a chance to grow in the first place.

The goal of my plan is not to deny you food; it's to replace the abundance of carbs in your diet with low-carb alternatives. We have examples in the back of the book, and you can also find low-carb alternatives online. There are a lot of options out there.

No doubt, weight loss is hard. But as I've said, keeping it off is even harder, which is why—and I repeat—80 percent of the people who lose weight gain it back. That's why I wrote this book. Any number of fad diets can help you lose weight. This book will help you understand what is happening in your body when you eat certain foods and help you build long-term strategies and habits to help you keep the weight off. The first part of the book is like preparing the cabin as you come in for a smooth landing (Phases 1 and 2). By the time you touch down to your goal weight, you are ready to cruise to success (Phase 3, Maintenance).

Unfortunately, the medical profession basically lets patients treat obesity on their own. A recent study (The Action Study) stated that 82 percent of patients feel that treating obesity is their responsibility alone. There are no other diseases that I can cite where doctors just look the other way when a patient comes in with all the symptoms. Imagine if patients were just handed a sheet of paper with a "suggested" meal plan if they had diabetes or hypertension. Strokes, heart attacks, and amputations would be even more common than they already are. In some ways, that's what the profession is doing with obesity. The medical profession needs to recognize and treat obesity as a disease. And we must do so, using the guidelines that our national organizations have laid out for us. Based on the science, many of them tout the merits of a low-carb diet.

A low-carb diet is transformative. It will change your life, as it has changed mine. You will lose the weight without going hungry, you will look more fit, and you will feel healthier and likely happier than you have in a long time.

The Benefits of Getting to a Healthier Weight with the No Guesswork Plan

I told you (and will continue to go over) all the bad things that can happen with obesity, but I didn't give you a synopsis of all the good things that are going to happen to you when you get to a healthier weight. Getting to a healthier weight is not about appearance. Getting to a healthier weight (particularly with the NGW plan) is about all the many health benefits such as:

- Helping with fertility (I actually have to warn couples about this so they don't get a surprise in 9 months)
- Helping relieve pain from arthritis
- Decreasing risk of heart disease
- Getting rid of/better control of: diabetes, high blood pressure, polycystic ovarian syndrome (PCOS), among many other medical conditions
- Boosting your immune system
- Reducing inflammation
- Boosting energy
- Extending your lifespan
- Improving depression and anxiety
- And many, many, more health benefits

I could go on and on, but I wanted to just give you a few of the many benefits that will happen to you once you get to a healthier weight. We will talk about many of them throughout this book but I wanted to give you a preview of what you have to look forward to. You are ready, now let's get started!

CHAPTER FOUR

The Mindset for Change

A former college football player, whom I will call Carl, came to see me in early 2018 for treatment of severe back pain. He had been fit in school, but years of eating fast food regularly had turned his once-muscular build into one with obesity. He also had been diagnosed with sleep apnea just a few weeks prior. Now in his mid-thirties, Carl needed to lose weight to get rid of the pain and sleep disorder. His diet was heavy with carbs—bread, French fries, soft drinks, sweets, and more. So, I asked him to focus on making one simple, consistent change (OSCC): to reduce his consumption of carbs to below 100 grams a day (with a target of 75 grams). That's it for now, I told him.

To meet that criteria, Carl mostly would have to eat meats (without batter or sauces), leafy green vegetables, eggs, cheese, and healthy fats, but he could have as much of those foods as he needed to feel satisfied, I explained. He didn't have to count calories, measure portions, or eat pre-packaged foods. He listened intently and assured me he would give it a try. A month later, when he returned for his checkup, Carl had lost twenty pounds! I was astonished, and he seemed surprised that I was so surprised.

"I just did what you told me, doc," he said. "And I'm not hungry!"

Patients don't always do exactly what I ask. But Carl was ready to change.

Another of my patients, a woman in her mid- to late 60s, came to see me for multiple health issues. Weighing in at more than 350 pounds, she had significant swelling in her legs, similar to elephantiasis, and her legs were "weeping," releasing a clear fluid, like tears. She felt horrible because she hadn't been able to lose weight. She walked with a cane and could barely move. She wore slippers because her feet could no longer fit her shoes. Like many of my patients, she had been told she needed to eat less and exercise more. When she first came into my program, I told her the same thing I tell most of my new patients: Make one simple, consistent change (OSCC): keep her consumption of carbs to below 100 grams per day (with a target of 75 grams). She did that, and within the first three to four weeks, she lost twenty pounds, much of the weight loss coming from her legs. She was overjoyed that she could finally put on shoes again. She, too, was ready to change. In fact, when she came to me, she was already in Stage Three of what psychological research tells us are the five distinct stages of change. Psychologists Carlo DiClemente and James O. Prochaska conducted the study, which involved 872 people who were trying to change their smoking habits. The study identified five stages that became known as the Transtheoretical Model of Change. The stages are:

1. **Pre-contemplation**, when people do not plan to change in the near future or may not be even aware that change is needed.
2. **Contemplation**, when people are aware that change is needed and plan to do something in the near future (within the next six months), but they are weighing the pros and cons.
3. **Preparation**, when people are ready for change and plan to take action within the next month.
4. **Action**, when people have taken action to modify their behavior to achieve a desired result.
5. **Maintenance**, when people have changed their behavior and are working to maintain it and prevent a relapse.

My goal is to reach people in the Pre-contemplation and Contemplation stages and persuade them to change their lifestyles. The sooner I can persuade them of the health benefits and relative ease of the low-carb lifestyle, the sooner they will be on their way to a healthier and hopefully happier life. Many who enter my program are just not sure they can do it. By the time they get to me, they have tried multiple times to lose weight on their own (an average of about ten or more times), they've tried various commercial weight loss plans, and they've tried other, less comprehensive medical weight loss plans. They often feel like a failure. They feel ashamed, dejected, and hopeless. Perhaps you are in the same place. Like the first meeting with my patients, this chapter is all about helping you to change your mindset. Obesity is not your fault. It's not just about willpower. In Chapter Three we talked about how your own body can work against you. Perhaps you've been blaming yourself all these years. Well, the blame alone is enough to make it difficult to change your mindset. Take a deep breath and feel that burden of guilt lifting from you. Allow yourself to believe again. Now, you are ready to change.

Often, patients come to me already in the Preparation stage, already ready to change, especially when health issues push them to get the help they need, like the woman with the weeping legs. Sometimes, they are just tired of being miserable, like the former football player. The quick weight loss he achieved helped to boost his confidence that he could really change his life. Whether or not he realized it, he was already well on his way.

One of the most important first steps in changing your life is a positive mindset. That's why I want to spend a little time on the subject before we get into the details of how my program works. Think of the many clichés you've heard about the power of positive thinking and believing in yourself, sayings like, "If you believe, you can achieve." Remember the children's story, "The Little Engine That Could"? *I think I can, I think I can, I think I can*...There's more to it than just "feel good psychology." Countless studies have shown the correlation between a positive mindset and a positive outcome. Medical researchers have seen this phenomenon with the so-called "placebo effect," where many patients in clinical trials report improvement in their symptoms, even if they were administered only a sugar pill or other inactive substance in place of real medication. They expected to feel better, so they did. A study by Fabrizio Benedetti, a physiology and neuroscience professor at the University of Turin, even documented measurable biological improvements when patients expected to receive an effective treatment, even if they received only fake drugs. Their expectation of success was key.

Dr. Alia Crum, a psychologist from Stanford University, followed a group of women who worked as housekeepers as part of a study testing the power of mindset. She asked the housekeepers (who of course spent the day laboring on their feet) a simple question: "Do you exercise regularly?" The majority of the women (two-thirds) responded that they did not. She measured the women—their weight and body fat—and asked questions about their satisfaction with their jobs. They were then split into two groups. Half of the women were given a fifteen-minute presentation, showing that their work was a good source of exercise. The presentation even detailed how many calories they were likely burning as part of their regular work day. The other group was not given such a presentation. Four weeks later, the women were measured again. The women who had been given the presentation experienced a reduction of their weight, body fat, and blood pressure, while the other group saw no measurable change.

Dr. Crum conducted a similar study with two groups of university students, who were told they were drinking either a decadent milkshake or a fat-free, diet one. The students were tested, and in those who thought they were drinking the traditional, fattening milkshake, the hormone that signals to the brain that you are hungry (ghrelin) had decreased significantly. This, of course, made them feel full (i.e. not hungry). But the students who thought they were drinking the diet shake saw no significant decrease in their hunger hormone level, and thus they still felt the same amount of hunger. The truth is that all of the students had been given the exact same drink. It was their mindset that controlled how their bodies responded.

As I mentioned, many of the patients who seek treatment at my weight management clinic have tried just about everything to lose weight, but they always ended up in the same frustrating place. Why? In their minds, they were on a diet. Translation: Something temporary. So, when they returned to their usual eating habits, the weight came back. My program is a **lifestyle change**. So the diet is not temporary, it's a diet for life. If you understand and accept that high level of commitment from the beginning, it can make all the difference in your success.

Author Daniel Coyle explores this phenomenon in his book, *The Talent Code: Greatness Isn't Born. It's Grown. Here's How.* In it, he shares the story of Professor Gary McPherson, who decided in 1997 to study why some children progress more quickly at music lessons than others. McPherson randomly selected 157 children and tracked their progress from a few weeks before they chose their instrument to their high school graduation. He videotaped their practices and conducted detailed interviews with them. One of the first questions McPherson asked was this: "How long do you think you'll play your new instrument?" The students were given the following options: through this year, through primary school, through high school, or all my life. The children's responses were grouped into three categories: short-term commitment, medium commitment, or long-term commitment. Then McPherson grouped the amount of time each child practiced as follows: low (twenty minutes per week), medium (forty-five minutes per week), and high (ninety minutes per week). When McPherson plotted the results against the students' performance on a skills test, the results were stunning. With the same amount of practice, the students in the long-term commitment group outperformed the short-term commitment students by 400 percent. Even with just twenty minutes of practice per week, the long-term commitment group progressed faster than the short-term commitment students who practiced for one and a half hours.

Somehow, the most successful students had latched onto the notion that music was something they could do for the rest of their lives, and that belief propelled them to the top of the heap. "What ignited the progress wasn't any innate skill or gene," Coyle wrote. "It was a small, ephemeral, yet powerful idea: a vision of their ideal future selves, a vision that oriented, energized and accelerated progress..." Those who had the mindset and the highest time commitment did even better. Just imagine what you could do if you had the same mindset and the same commitment to get to a healthier weight.

Physicians usually don't like to focus on this part of weight management (the mindset part). They jump right into the program, telling the patients what they can and cannot eat, prescribing medicines, and giving orders to exercise. Then, they schedule a follow-up visit to see if the patient is actually losing weight. But I know on a personal level the importance of mindset in achieving a goal. I know how important it is to have a mindset geared for change to achieve what appears to be an insurmountable goal. And I know how crucial this step is to achieve any long-term success. It's the most critical part.

When I was in high school, two of my best friends and I latched onto an idea that we could become doctors together. We had grown up in the roughest parts of Newark, New Jersey, in broken families, with no father figures, with drugs and desperation all around us. The streets almost snared us. But because we believed (with the help of our counselor) that we could one day become doctors, three African American boys who statistics said most likely would wind up in jail or dead stuck together and instead managed to accomplish what seemed impossible. We became doctors (fondly known as The Three Doctors); one of my friends is an emergency room physician and the other is a dentist, assistant dean, and dental school professor. We couldn't have done it without a long-term commitment and without our heads in the game. For you to accomplish your goal of losing weight and keeping it off, you have to have your head in the game. And you need a mindset geared for change.

For one of my patients, a vision of his future also ignited a long-term commitment to change his life, but in his case it was a vision of what he did *not* want to become. He weighed over 400 pounds when he visited a sick co-worker in the hospital. His co-worker was a little older, with severe obesity, and suffered from an array of health issues. My patient looked at his colleague lying in the hospital bed, struggling to stay alive, and saw himself fifteen years down the road, which he realized wasn't that far away. He saw a future he did not want and decided then that he would do what he could to lose the weight and keep it off. And that's exactly what he did. He made a long-term commitment to change his life, and that commitment helped to catapult him to success.

Two important questions I always ask my patients are:

1. Do you think this is a plan you can maintain? (because remember what I said, if you go back to eating the same way you have always eaten, you will go back to the same weight you always were.) This is a lifestyle designed for you to stick to for the rest of your life.
2. After trying a low-carb diet for a while, are you convinced that this plan works? If so, that's half the battle. Even if you stumble from time to time, you know which diet/lifestyle works to get you to a healthy weight. That's better than going out there trying the next fad diet after the next fad diet, ending up in an endless loop of failed dieting.

Writer James Clear, who studies habits, goal-setting, and change, says the key to changing behavior for good is to create an identity that drives your performance. He calls this "identity-based habits." In other words, you first have to believe that you are the kind of person who can achieve the change you desire before you set any goals. If you believe, for example, that you are a determined person, your actions toward a specific goal will line up with what you believe about yourself. You are more likely to make decisions that show you are determined to meet your goal. It would be of little value to set a goal of losing twenty pounds if you believe you are the type of person who can't stick to anything. Your belief about yourself can become a self-fulfilling prophecy. Even if your past has shown that you have difficulty being consistent, it is possible to create a new identity. Even more, you are more likely to lose those twenty pounds if you change how you think about yourself. First, as Clear says, you have to decide the type of person you want to become, and then take small steps towards becoming that person. If, for example, you want to be a person who eats few carbs, make yourself a low-carb breakfast, or choose grilled chicken, veggies, and salad for lunch and repeat the behavior, taking small steps towards becoming the person you want to be (remember my mantra, OSCC- One Simple Consistent Change). Remember, things are connected. If you make One Simple Consistent Change (OSCC), that change is connected to at least five other things, and when the one thing you've changed moves, it moves the other things connected to it. So if that change moves in a negative direction, all the things connected move in a negative direction as well, but if it moves in a positive direction, then all the things connected to that One Simple Consistent Change (OSCC) move in a positive direction. I know it can be daunting to look all the way down the road. Don't worry about that right now, start with OSCC- Once Simple Consistent Change. Focus on that first, becoming the kind of *person* you want to become with just One Simple Consistent Change, instead of focusing on the pounds you want to lose. This way, it will be easier to begin with focusing on just that one thing, and thus your commitment will be greater. Soon you will see other things change that are connected to your One Simple Consistent Change and you will start to see your success unfold right in front of you.

Finally, before we jump into the details of how my program works, I also want to remind you to be patient with yourself. Even with the right mindset, it takes time to change. It takes time for the new lifestyle behaviors you will develop to become automatic. Forget the myth that it takes twenty-one days to change a habit. That misconstrued notion has lingered since 1960, when a plastic surgeon named Maxwell Maltz described in a best-selling book that it often took his patients a *minimum* of twenty-one days to get used to seeing a new face in the mirror or to get accustomed to life without an arm or leg. That critical word, *minimum,* got lost in the translation, and we have been told ever since by many in the self-help industry that all it takes to change our bad habits if we are committed is twenty-one days. It's a no-brainer why people would latch onto that idea. Twenty-one days is just three short weeks! Who wouldn't want to be able to change a bad habit in just three weeks? But researchers have shown that changing behavior or forming a new habit actually takes much longer.

One such researcher was Phillippa Lally, who conducted a study in 2009 at the University College London to figure out just how long it takes to form a habit, and she then published her findings in the *European Journal of Social Psychology.* Lally and her research team studied ninety-six people over a period of twelve weeks. Each person selected just one new habit for that time frame. The choices ranged from drinking a bottle of water with lunch to running for fifteen minutes before dinner. They reported each day on whether they did the behavior that they chose and how automatic it felt. At the end of the study, the research team analyzed the results and found that on average it took sixty-six days—more than two months—for the new behavior to feel automatic. But the results ranged widely from eighteen days to 254 days (well past the initial study period in some cases). Plus, the researchers found that if the subject missed one opportunity to perform the behavior, it didn't substantially change the process of forming a habit. The takeaway lessons from that study are:

1. It may take *up to* eight months of consistent behavior—or less for some of you—for the changes you are making to feel automatic, so be patient with yourself.
2. Even if you slip off track but quickly get back on it, you can still

change your behavior in the same time frame. Consistency is key. (Remember, OSCC, One Simple Consistent Change.) Those who were inconsistent were not successful in forming a habit.

Even when you are mentally ready to change—you are motivated, you have a positive mindset, and you are committed to changing your life for the long haul—change is still hard. Part of that is because we do much of what we do mindlessly. Which is why the practice of *mindfulness* is so important. Studies show that about 40 percent of people's daily activities are performed every single day in almost the same way with little thought. In other words, 40 percent of the time, we're doing things without even thinking much—or at all—about what we are doing. This behavior is based on habits we've developed over time. We were likely *mindful* about these behaviors at first, deciding to do something a certain way at a certain time because it worked for our lives. Then, after months, maybe years, of doing it the same way, our minds perform that behavior in the same context on autopilot. For example, if you start a new job, you have to figure out what time you have to leave home to get to work on time and the route you're going to take to get there. Initially, you may have to try different routes to figure out which is best, but once you figure that out and begin doing the same thing the same way, day after day, it becomes automatic. How many times have you thrown clothes in the car planning to stop at the dry cleaner on the way to work, but then you drive directly to the office and, at the end of the day, when you're about to get back into the car to head home, you get a glimpse of your suit still on the back seat? This happens to me because when I get in the car at the same time each morning, my brain is basically programmed to go straight to work. The clothes in the back seat are out of sight, as my mind shifts to autopilot.

Professor Wendy Wood, Provost Professor of Psychology and Business at the University of Southern California, has conducted extensive studies of habits. She says we develop the kind of habitual behaviors discussed above based on "associative learning." We associate one activity with another or with a certain place or thing, for example; eating popcorn at the movie. If we always eat popcorn at the movie theater, the cinema becomes a cue for eating popcorn. Wood and a team of researchers conducted a study, using popcorn, to determine which factors disrupt and maintain habit performance. The study participants were given popcorn to eat under a variety of different circumstances, and people who always ate popcorn at the cinema were not influenced by whether they were hungry or how much they liked the popcorn. When inside the cinema, they ate equal amounts of stale and fresh popcorn. They ate out of habit, but only in the context associated with that past behavior (the cinema) and only when allowed to eat the way they usually did in the past (with their dominant hand). "The thoughtful intentional mind is easily derailed and people tend to fall back on habitual behaviors. Forty percent of the time we're not thinking about what we're doing," Dr. Wood said in 2014, during her session at the American Psychological Association's 122nd Annual Convention in Washington, D.C. "Habits allow us to focus on other things...Willpower is a limited resource, and when it runs out, you fall back on habits."

So, then, what are some practical steps to developing new habits? Wood identifies three key principles to changing old habits and forming new ones:

1. **Derail existing habits by disrupting the way you usually do things.** Wood calls this a "window of opportunity" to act on your new intentions. So, if your goal is to cut the carbs from your diet, you have to restock and rearrange your pantry and refrigerator with low-carb options. That will disrupt the thoughtless habit of grabbing a bag of potato chips, cookies or soft drink when you want a snack. Also, if by chance you are starting a new job or moving to a new house or new city, that's an excellent opportunity to change the habits connected to those "cues."
2. **Repeat. Repeat. Repeat.** As mentioned earlier, there is no substitute for repeating the new behavior you want to develop. And you have to do so consistently (remember my mantra OSCC) for a period that could stretch anywhere from a few weeks to up to eight months for the behavior to feel automatic. Did I mention that this requires patience?

3. **Use stable context cues to trigger a new pattern of behavior.** It's much easier to develop a new pattern of behavior if it is connected to something we do regularly already. For example, if you want to start walking more every day, you can decide that you are going to begin walking for a half-hour every day after lunch, and you repeat that behavior. Over time, eating lunch becomes a trigger for walking.

These are great tips for developing healthy habits. But habitual behavior is a state of mindlessness. We don't have to think about what we're doing; we just do it because we are accustomed to doing it that way. When it comes to eating, I encourage my patients to be *mindful* as often as possible. Mindfulness is a mental state achieved by focusing on the present moment, acknowledging and accepting your feelings, thoughts, and bodily sensations. It is the exact opposite of auto-pilot. Mindful eating is:

- Allowing yourself to become aware of the positive and nurturing opportunities that are available through food selection and preparation.
- Using all your senses (acknowledging taste, smell, appearance) in choosing to eat food that is both satisfying to you and nourishing to your body.
- Acknowledging responses to food (likes, dislikes, or neutral) without judgment.
- Becoming aware of physical hunger and satiety cues to guide your decisions to begin and end eating. Take time to taste your food and savor its look, flavor, and smell. Pay attention to cues for when you are satisfied; don't just continue to eat until you feel stuffed. In the same way it takes your brain twenty minutes to slow down your limbic system (i.e. cravings), it also takes your brain twenty minutes to know your stomach is full (i.e. physically stretched). A good example of this is Thanksgiving. You stuff your face with all the great food that's in front of you and then twenty minutes later, you are sitting on the couch with that uncomfortable feeling in your stomach because you ate too much. That's why I tell my patients to eat half as much as they would normally eat, but eat it over a 20-minute period. That way you've only eaten half as much but still feel just as full. Not only

that, but your limbic system (i.e. cravings) will slow down over that twenty-minute period as well. Try it out, you'll see. A trick to doing this is to eat your meal in courses. The patient who lost the most in my program (230 pounds) did this. But he could only do it at dinner because of his busy schedule. He would have his salad first, enjoy that with his water, and when he was done, he would get up and put that in the sink. Next he would eat his soup, enjoy that, then get up and put the bowl in the sink. And then finally he would have his main meal, which was half of what he had eaten since he already had a soup and salad. Doing it that way would take him at least twenty minutes. And he found not only was he just as full as if he had eaten double the amount in five minutes, but the meal was even more enjoyable than before because he had something to look forward to next. So, after his salad, he looked forward to enjoying his soup and then after the soup he had his main meal to look forward to. It's just a little trick you can try to extend your meal to twenty minutes. Also, don't forget to put the fork down between every bite. That will also help extend your mealtime.

- Understanding the difference between hunger and craving. This may seem trivial, but it often trips people up. Hunger is the feeling that your stomach is empty, and you need to fill it. You experience almost a physical need for food. Craving is different and can pop up even when your stomach is full. You want to eat a particular food, not to fill your stomach, but because you either thought about, saw (temptation, which is another form of craving) or smelled it and have become fixated on it. Sometimes, hunger and craving co-exist, which is the worst combination. It is why I recommend that you never go to the supermarket on an empty stomach. If you are hungry, you are more likely to see tempting foods that trigger cravings.

Finally, I want to remind you about your reset button, another one of my mantras. I was reminded of it one morning as I woke up to get ready for work. That annoying beep of my alarm clock woke me up at 5:30 a.m. I wasn't quite ready to jump out of bed, so I reached over and hit the snooze button. As I lay there with my eyes open, a thought popped in my mind: Today is a new day. Just like I hit that snooze button, I can hit the reset button on life when things don't take off exactly as I expected. That is one of the most beautiful things in life. Every morning you wake up, you get a chance to hit the reset button. You get another day to work on your goals or make the changes in life you've always wanted to make. Feel good about the fact that you don't have to repeat yesterday. So, when you open your eyes in the morning, smile, take a deep breath, slowly exhale, reach over, and then, if needed, hit that reset button and make today the best day ever.

CHAPTER 5

PHASE ONE
#WhatsYourCarbNumber

Now you've reached the heart of this book: how the No Guesswork (NGW) Plan works. And it's time to do what you've been promising yourself you would do. As you know, time flies. Before you know it, another year will be gone. So don't procrastinate another day. Let's get started...NOW!

As a physician, I must remind you to consult your doctor before starting any weight management plan, including this one. I have guided many of my own patients in achieving great results with this plan, and I am confident the same can happen for you. But your doctor knows your particular medical issues and may want to monitor you, especially if you have diabetes, high blood pressure, or heart disease. That's important because your weight loss may be so rapid that your medications soon may need adjusting. Don't be surprised, though, if your doctor tries to push a low-fat diet on you. Many doctors still don't understand the science of weight management. They bought into the low-fat hype (a fifty-year experiment that has repeatedly failed) and now are resistant to the truth about the health benefits of a low-carb lifestyle. But you are the best advocate for your health, and so feel free to share this book with your doctor so that he or she will know the source of your information (a physician who practices obesity medicine!). My book also will help your doctor understand more about the lifestyle change you are making.

Remember the 6 S's? It's the basis of my program: Simple, Safe, Sustainable, Satisfying, Superior, and Sugarless. The approach is a low-carb one, though not necessarily a keto approach. So, what's the difference between my plan and the keto diet that is getting so much attention? NGW is personalized just for you, and it permits most of you to eat more carbs (than you would with keto), which expands your meal possibilities. Let me explain. A low-carb diet is defined as a meal plan that recommends eating fewer than 150 grams of total carbs per day. A keto diet generally sets the limit at 50 grams of total carbs per day. My plan recognizes that not all bodies work the same, and so the maximum number of carbs a person can eat and still lose weight is individual. My plan helps you find your individual "carb number." Some of you may choose to keep your carbs under 50 grams per day for quicker results, and that is absolutely fine. But Phase One of my plan helps you find your custom number, and if you stay beneath that number, you will lose an average of one to two pounds per week.

That's the goal of Phase One: for you to lose an average of one to two pounds per week until you lose 10 percent of your current weight. Why 10 percent? Between 5 percent and 10 percent is the amount of weight loss needed to yield what the medical community considers "clinically meaningful." That is the amount of weight that you need to lose to see improvements in medical conditions, such as diabetes, hypertension, arthritis, blood pressure, sleep apnea, etc. A 10 percent reduction in weight also will likely result in a reduction of medications for those who are on them. I chose the higher goal (10 percent) because NGW yields significant results. Once you find your personalized carb number, you can achieve that 10 percent weight loss goal and more.

So #WhatsYourCarbNumber?

This step sets NGW apart from other low-carb programs out there. Our bodies are all different, and they metabolize food at different rates. While one person may be able to eat slightly more carbs than average and lose weight, another might have to eat fewer carbs to lose the same amount of weight. My plan helps you figure out what works for you. The good news is that you can start wherever you are. You don't have to feel guilty anymore. It's not your fault if you are struggling to lose weight. Regardless of what you've been told throughout your life, obesity is not just about willpower. As you now know, your body can work against you when you're trying to lose weight. Knowledge is power. So let's use that power to win this battle.

First Things First

We're about to get into the nuts and bolts of the NGW plan, but there are some things you will need to do to prepare. First, I recommend you take a daily multivitamin, a probiotic, and a fish oil capsule if you don't eat fish at least once to twice per week. You will get most of the nutrients you need from your low-carb meals, but a multivitamin assures that you get *all* of the important vitamins and minerals. Probiotics are basically "good bacteria" that help to keep the gut healthy and have been shown to aid in weight loss. And a fish oil tablet provides the important Omega-3 nutrients, which also have an array of health benefits. But the best (and tastiest) way to get the Omega-3's is to eat fish, particularly oily fish, such as salmon, once or twice a week. If you're allergic or just can't tolerate fish, though, the tablets are a good alternative. Once you have all of your supplements, put them in a place where you will remember to take them each day.

Next, you have to make a commitment to do two things: **track and plan**. People who track their meals do better, and people who plan do better. I'm not telling you what I think, read, or heard. I'm telling you what I know firsthand. I've studied the science, and I treat patients every day. But better yet, I'm living it. I do this myself, and I know it works.

Let's talk first about the importance of planning. Virtually everything we eat contains sugar and carbs, and all of the places where we get food, from restaurants to office parties, offer an overabundance of carbs. So, the only way to thrive with a low-carb lifestyle in this high-carb world is to plan. We will talk about this in more detail in a later chapter, but I want you to wrap your brain around this truth from the beginning. Planning may mean bringing your own "stuff," making your own lunches, checking out restaurant menus before going out to eat, bringing your own snacks to a party, or keeping your desk drawers and home pantries stocked with low-carb goodies. If you don't plan to succeed, you are almost assuredly setting yourself up to fail.

Tracking is just as important. It may seem tedious, but the ONLY way to find your carb number is to track. My NGW app helps make that process easier. Even after you've identified your carb number, tracking remains important. Without it, you are more than likely to underestimate the number of carbs in your diet and to overestimate your physical activity. It's human nature. A study I conducted shows this to be the case. But if you are keeping an accurate record of each meal and your physical activity in real time, you are much more likely to remember (and account for) every morsel that goes into your mouth, as well as the accurate amount of time you worked out.

A good tracker (often a mobile phone app) makes it easy for you to find the number of carbs in each food item. Tracking provides a reliable record that allows you to reflect on how well you are sticking to your goals; it also helps you figure out where you need improvement. Tracking holds you accountable to yourself and makes you more mindful of your eating and physical activity.

My patient Margaret, a fifty-something-year-old teacher, was compulsive about tracking in the beginning. Eventually, she began showing up for her appointments with spreadsheets, showing not only what she was eating, but her consistent weight loss over time. In less than a year, Margaret lost eighty pounds! She was super excited about how she looked and felt. For the first time in years, shopping was fun again. Then, she and her long-time boyfriend broke up. She stopped tracking. She started eating carbs again, and she regained thirty pounds. But no matter what, Margaret kept coming to her appointments. As long as she kept showing up, I knew there was hope. I recognized that she was depressed, and we got her some mental health counseling. Slowly, she became more stable and started tracking consistently again. And you know what? She started losing weight again.

Tracking keeps you honest. If you don't keep track of what you're putting in your mouth, you won't know for sure. Most of us tend to underestimate how much we eat, and eating without tracking is like spending money without knowing how much is in your bank account. I don't accept any excuses for not tracking. I don't want to hear you couldn't find every food item in the tracker or didn't have the time. Tracking is a commitment; there is no other way around it, you just have to do it. I have signs reminding patients when they get in my examination rooms to take out their phones so that I can see their trackers.

I can't tell you the number of times I've heard, "Doc, I'm not sure what's going on. I'm doing everything right. I'm doing the same thing I was doing before, but I'm not losing weight."

Me: "Are you tracking?"

Them: "Well, not like I was in the beginning…but I'm eating the same things, and I know my carbs are low."

Me: "Give me two weeks of consistent tracking. Track everything you put in your mouth."

Lo and behold, when they return two weeks later, they've lost weight. Their carbs weren't quite as low as they'd imagined when they weren't tracking. Honestly, the only way to know for sure is to track. A few carbs over your personalized number can shut down your weight loss completely. Newsflash: If your weight loss has stalled, there's always a reason, and it's not that the diet has stopped working for you. Consider this tip: If your personalized number is 70, stay well below 70, by at least 10 to 15 grams, to give yourself a little cushion. If you don't have time to track before you eat, at a minimum, take a picture of your plate to help you remember to track as soon as possible after your meal. The only other way to avoid tracking is to stay keto (under 50 grams of carbs, but closer to 20 grams per day) and eat only protein (chicken, fish, turkey, beef, pork), no batter or sauces, and non-starchy green veggies, and NOTHING else.

There are a number of helpful fitness apps for your mobile phone, such as MyFitnessPal, Lose It!, or my No Guesswork App to track your daily carb intake. The apps contain a daily food tracker that keeps tabs on everything you eat, and using them is a quick and easy process. You simply type in the name of the foods (including dishes from most restaurant chains), as well as the number of servings, and the app displays the number of carbs. The better apps also allow you to set daily goals for how many grams of carbs, fats, and proteins you want to eat and show after each meal how many you have left before exceeding your goal. My No Guesswork app focuses on keeping your carbs down and is designed to make it easy for you to follow my program.

Once you've downloaded the app, you're ready to get started.

Step One—Cutting The Carbs

A diet is generally considered low-carb if it requires eating less than 150 carbs per day. But the vast majority of people (80 percent) won't lose weight unless they reduce their carbs to fewer than 100 grams a day. A small percentage of people (about 10 to 15 percent) have to get below 50 grams of carbs per day to lose weight; that's the basis of the keto approach. And virtually 100 percent of people will lose weight if they get below 30 grams per day. It would seem then that 30 is the magic number. So, why not just require everyone to restrict their carbs to less than 30 grams per day? Well, I like to flip that logic. Why restrict everybody to 30 grams of carbs a day, when the vast majority of people can lose weight without having to reduce their carbs by that much? That's what the NGW plan is all about: individuality. We will find your individual number. We want to make this lifestyle as easy as possible (remember the 6 S's), so I don't want to be any more restrictive than necessary.

For starters, I want you to aim to get your average daily carb intake below 75 grams. That means you should strive to eat fewer than 75 grams of carbs per day. But remember, the fewer carbs you eat, the more weight you lose. So, if you're feeling really ambitious, you can aim for 50 grams of carbs per day.

I can't stress enough how important it is for you to stay at least below 75 grams of carbs. As few as 5 grams of carbs above your number (something as simple as an extra packet of ketchup) can cause your weight loss to stall. And yes, you must track everything, including condiments, like ketchup. Losing weight by reducing carbs is quite different than cutting calories to lose weight. In a low-calorie approach, you can lose a little bit of weight if you restrict your calories by a little bit. And if you restrict your calories a lot, you can lose a lot of weight. It doesn't work that way with carbs. If you restrict your carbs a little bit (say from 300 grams per day down to 200 grams per day), you still likely won't lose any weight. Even if you restrict your carbs by a lot (say from 300 grams per day all the way down to 100 grams per day), you still may not lose any weight if you didn't reach your carb number. It doesn't matter that you cut your carbs by a third. You have to get below your *personalized* carb number or drop below an average of 50 grams of carbs per day (ketosis) to lose weight.

Your goal of 75 carbs is like having 75 cents to spend. You can spend that 75 cents however you like, but remember, you only have 75 cents. So if you want to blow it on a bag of chips, you can do that, but it wouldn't be wise. That bag might cost you 50 cents, leaving you only 25 cents to spend for the rest of the day. Get it? If you plan wisely, the majority of your carbs should come from your vegetables. There will be other miscellaneous carbs in sauces and salads, etc. that will make up the rest of your carbs.

What Can I Eat?

This is probably *the* most asked question. And the short answer is a lot of good stuff. Among the advantages of the low-carb lifestyle is that you don't have to deal with hunger at any point. A low-calorie diet requires you to eat less and less to keep losing weight and to maintain it (I call that semi-starvation). But you can enjoy the same healthy portions from beginning to end under my program. So be creative. The meal options are plentiful — all kinds of meats, non-starchy vegetables, and fats (yes, fats!). But stay away from all refined carbohydrates, including breads, rice, pasta, potatoes, and sugar (yes, that means most desserts!). They will sabotage your success. However, there are many low-carb desserts that you can enjoy and still stay on track. Some recipes are included in the back of the book, and you can find an array of good choices online.

Think of it this way: Every scoop of rice is a scoop of sugar. Every fork of pasta is a scoop of sugar. And every piece of bread is four scoops of sugar! You also will have to limit your consumption of certain fruits; a banana, for example, contains as many carbs as a Snickers bar. Even though the banana is naturally sweet, the body can't distinguish the sugar in that banana from the sugar in a candy bar. But berries have fewer grams of carbohydrates and can work in a low-carb meal plan. So, in Phase One and Phase Two, I recommend that the main fruits you eat are berries and avocados, but limit everything else.

Your meals should be built around proteins and fats. Meats and seafood, which are high in protein, have zero carbs, but watch the added sauces and condiments, which can contain high amounts of carbs in small amounts. For example, one tablespoon of ketchup is 5 grams of carbs; two tablespoons of barbeque sauce, 12 carbs. But one tablespoon of butter, which is high in fat, has zero carbs, as does one tablespoon of olive oil. As a rule of thumb, if it (whatever it is) tastes sweet, it's probably loaded with sugar.

Fortunately, the growing popularity of low-carb programs has created a demand for more quick, low-carb options, and the market is responding (albeit slowly) with low-carb alternatives to such staples as spaghetti (spaghetti squash or thin, spiraled zucchini), rice (riced cauliflower), and even tater tots (veggie tots). But be careful of pre-packaged foods, even if they are advertised as low-carb. They often are higher in carbs than you might think. Read the labels carefully to determine their carb content. Over time, you will get good at knowing how many carbs are in certain foods. You will eventually become a carb-ologist (what I call someone who can tell you the amount of carbs in just about any food)!

What about ultra-processed or processed foods, like bacon? They're not ideal, but bacon would be better than others that contain sugar and refined carbs. So, enjoy some of them for now, if they help in your transition to a low-carb lifestyle. Bottom line is, read the label for carb content. The goal is to get you to a healthy weight and eliminate the health ailments associated with obesity. But as we transition into the Maintenance Phase, we will slowly limit the processed/ultra-processed foods and move to a more low-carb, Mediterranean-style diet that adds a few more healthy carbs (like complex carbs, such as fiber-rich foods). For the time being, though, eat what you enjoy — as long as it enables you to stay under your carb number. Remember a potato is not a processed food, it is a whole food, but if a person with diabetes ate three to four potatoes a day, their sugar would rise to dangerous levels. So the bottom line is watch your carb content and shift to a low-carb Mediterranean diet as you progress through the program. Just so you know what is considered ultra-processed food. In short, ultra-processed food is any food in a package or can. Examples of ultra-processed foods are: carbonated soft drinks, sweet, salty snacks, bread, buns, and biscuits, cookies, pastries, cakes, margarine, sweetened cereals, fruit yogurts, energy drinks, packaged soups, noodles and deserts, fish and chicken nuggets or sticks, sausage, burgers, hot dogs, and other reconstituted meat products. But again, the bottom line is, watch the carb content as we transition to a low-carb Mediterranean diet.

Don't forget to rely on your tracking app. It will be your best friend, but like most friends, it's not perfect. So, if the amount of carb grams listed for a food item seems too good to be true, it probably is. But you can cross-reference the carb content listed in the app with another app or look for the food's nutritional information found online. If the app underestimates the food you are eating by 10 to 20 grams per day, your weight loss might stall. Use your app to explore how many carbs are in the foods you love, and if the numbers are too high, figure out an alternative. There's usually a delicious alternative; you just have to think creatively. The back of this book contains an array of meal ideas and even food swap suggestions to help in the process.

Finding Your Carb Number

While it is vitally important that you stay under the daily average of 75 grams of carbs during the first two weeks, don't panic if you go over 75 grams of carbs one day. Simply reduce your carbs even more the next day so that the weekly average is below 75 grams.

In the example below, Saturday was a bad day. The patient consumed 120 grams of carbs but quickly got back on track, significantly reducing his or her carbs (to 30 grams) the next day. So, the daily average that week was 70, below the goal of 75. If you're using the NGW app, it does the work, calculating your daily carb average each week. But to do it on your own, just add the total number of carb grams you ate each day for the entire first week and divide by seven.

Day of the Week	Total Carbs
Monday	70g
Tuesday	60
Wednesday	65
Thursday	70
Friday	75
Saturday	120
Sunday	30
Total carbs	490
Average (490 ÷7)	70

After the first week, it's time to weigh yourself. Pick your day. You should weigh yourself each week on the *same day, the same way.* You can weigh yourself more frequently if you like but the "official weigh-in" should be weekly. If you started on Sunday with a weigh-in, then Sunday is the day to record your weight each week. I recommend you weigh yourself in the morning, in your birthday suit, after your trip to the bathroom, and you should always follow that routine — same day, same way! I also recommend getting a Bluetooth scale that measures body composition, as well as weight. There are a variety of brands on the market, and they tend to be a bit expensive (around $100), but it's a good investment. Later, you will be asked to track your muscle mass to make sure you are not losing muscle, and a body composition scale enables you to do that. But if you cannot afford to buy a new scale, don't let that be an excuse to delay your fresh start. Work with what you have. After you weigh, enter your weight manually into your fitness tracker. Again, some of the fitness apps, like the NGW app, can be synced with your Bluetooth scale, and the data from the scale is recorded automatically in the app each week.

Repeat the same steps for the second week — enjoying delicious foods, eating when you're hungry, planning, and tracking everything you put in your mouth from drinks to mints. Now it's time to weigh again for the second week. Have you lost one to two pounds per week each week (at least two to four pounds)? If so, that's great! Let's figure out your number.

I know you were shooting to stay under 75 grams per week, but what was your actual daily average of carb grams those two weeks? You can figure it out in one or two easy ways. First, if you already determined your weekly daily average for Weeks One and Two, just add those two figures and divide by two. Let's say your average daily carb grams for the first week was 70, and then 74 for the second week (Step one: 70 + 74 = 144; Step two: 144 ÷ 2 = 72). Or, another way to do it is to add your actual carb grams for each day and divide by 14. (If your total for each of the 14 days equals 1008, then 1008 ÷ 14 = 72) Either way, voilà! You now know your personal carb number. In the example above, this person's carb number is 72! So in other words, this person would need to stay at or below 72 grams of carbs per day on average for the week in order to lose one to two pounds per week. And to play it safe, I recommend staying even 5 to 10 grams below that number (so the "safe" number would be an average between 67 and 62 carbs per week). Got it?

Now, we have to test that number. (If you didn't lose weight the first two weeks, don't be discouraged. We will not leave you behind. Skip to the next section about what to do if you didn't lose weight.) To test your number, just be diligent about keeping your carbs below your personal number for two more weeks. If, for example, your number is 72, make sure your daily average is under 72 grams. If you continue to lose one to two pounds over the next two weeks, congratulations, we cracked the code! You know your carb number for sure, and that will be your personal number until you've reached your weight loss goal and move to the maintenance phase, when you can add a few more carbs back to your diet. It's smooth sailing for you from here. Just keep repeating what you've been doing.

But wait! What if you thought you had found your carb number when you lost weight the first two weeks, but then you didn't lose weight the next two weeks? Don't panic! The next section is for you. (If you've found your carb number and confirmed it, you can skip the next section.)

Help! My Weight Loss Stopped Or I Didn't Lose Any Weight — Now What?

If your excitement over losing two to four pounds the first two weeks quickly turned to disappointment when your weight loss stalled the second two weeks, take a deep breath. You most likely didn't do anything wrong. The initial weight loss was likely just water weight. Your carb number was low enough to get rid of excess water but not quite low enough to burn the fat. We just have to make a slight adjustment.

What if you didn't lose even a pound a week the first two weeks? Let's pause to reflect for a moment. Are you absolutely sure that you tracked everything (and I do mean everything!) and that you kept your average daily carb number below 75 for both weeks? If you missed the mark in some way, don't be hard on yourself. This is a no-judgment zone. Just wipe the slate clean and start anew (remember what I said: you can always hit the reset button). Try again to get your average daily carbs under 75 grams, and let's see what happens. But if you tracked diligently and kept your average daily carbs under 75 grams, yet you still didn't lose weight, your carb number also was too high. In your case, too, we have to make an adjustment.

Here's the adjustment I want you to make if your experience is like one of the scenarios above: Decrease your average carb number by 10 grams. We reviewed earlier how to figure out your average daily carb grams for the first two weeks. So, if your number was 65, you now have to decrease that number by 10 and keep your carbs below 55 grams; if your average daily number of carbs the first two weeks was 70, you now drop to 60, and so on.

Try the new number for two weeks. Be sure that you are keeping your carbs below your new number. Again, weigh yourself each week — same day, same way. If you lost one to two pounds each week, then you, too, have found your number. Congratulations! This is the number that will help you reach your weight-loss goal. You are almost on cruise control. You will just have to test that number again for the next two weeks to confirm that this is indeed your number.

If you're losing more than one to two pounds per week, you are likely well below your carb number, and you can increase your weekly average by 10-gram increments until your weight loss is one to two pounds per week. But if you are doing fine there, you can keep going, knowing that your number is a little higher.

If you still haven't lost weight, I know you must be frustrated, but please don't give up. You are so close to getting the results that you desire. Our bodies all work differently, and you just happen to fall into that small group of people who have to get their carbs down to 50 grams or less to lose weight. Almost all people will lose weight if they keep their carbs on average below 50 grams. So that is your goal for the next two weeks: get below a daily average of 50 grams of carbs.

If getting below 50 grams of carbs didn't work (that's rarely the case), you will have to keep reducing your carbs every two weeks by 10 to 15 grams until you start losing weight. About 5 percent to 10 percent of people will have to get their carbs down to under 30 grams or less to lose weight. But once you get under an average of 30 carb grams, you are certain to get results.

Is decreasing your carbs that low dangerous? Not at all. It can be very healthy because to stay within your range, your diet will consist primarily of meats, fish, and leafy green vegetables. On the contrary, abdominal fat is dangerous to your health. Keeping your carbs low will help you lose fat, and losing fat is healthy. So, once you've kept your carbs below 30 grams for two weeks, and you're now losing weight, you, too, have found your carb number. Just figure out the daily average of carbs you consumed for those two weeks, and that's your number. You deserve much praise for hanging in there! The time and patience it took to get to this point were an investment in your future. You are on your way!

So, by now all of you should have your personalized carb number. This is your weight loss number for life. You will get a maintenance number later. But your weight loss number will help you change your life. Just for fun, compare numbers with your friends (#What'sYourCarbNumber). Join a movement of people who are achieving their weight loss and healthy-living goals with my plan. You can cruise through the first phase together. Phase One is about learning, exploring, and adapting to this low-carb life. You have learned what it takes for your body to lose weight, and you are working towards your weight goal. Explore different recipes and find foods you can enjoy the rest of your life. Discover what foods work well with your new lifestyle and what foods sabotage your weight loss. You've got this!

Remember, you will remain in Phase One until you've reached your 10 percent weight loss. Most people can accomplish that goal in three to four months. However, don't be discouraged if it takes you longer. Just keep working the plan, and it will work for you. So, let's recap:

1. Start off with a weekly average of 75 grams of carbs per day (meaning your daily average for the week should be 75 grams of carbs per day or less for the first two weeks). If you are losing weight at a rate of one to two pounds per week or more, then you most likely have found your number. Just figure out the average daily carbs you consumed over those two weeks, and that's your number.
2. Test that number for the next two weeks. If you continue losing weight, you've got your confirmation. You now have your customized carb number! If the weight loss stops, you only lost water weight,

and you need to decrease your number by another 10 grams. You should begin losing weight again.

3. If you haven't lost any weight at 75 grams, decrease your daily carb intake by 10 grams. Whatever your average daily carb intake was during those first two weeks, decrease it by 10 grams. You should see a weight loss of one to two pounds per week for the next two weeks. If you don't experience that rate of weight loss, continue to decrease your carbs by 10 grams every two weeks until you start to lose one to two pounds per week.
4. Once you find your number, stay there. Actually, I recommend staying at least 5 to 10 grams below that number to give yourself a little cushion until you complete Phase One (weight loss of 10 percent of your initial weight).
5. Remember: the goal is to keep your insulin low. And if your insulin is low, you burn fat! To keep your insulin low, you must keep your carbs low since carbs raise insulin.
6. If you're losing more than one to two pounds per week, you can increase your weekly average by 10-gram increments until your weight loss is one to two pounds per week.

Other Helpful Hints

Feed the Hunger Gremlin. Make sure the Hunger Gremlin (your ghrelin level) doesn't get to grow. The best way to do that is to eat a protein snack about an hour before your next meal. Even if you are not very hungry after eating your snack, you should eat something at meal time to keep that Gremlin at bay. If you get cravings at night, EAT! Just make sure you choose a protein or fat. They cost you nothing.

Do NOT count "net carbs!" Some low-carb programs subtract the fiber grams from the carbohydrates to get what is known as the "net carbs." About 75 to 80 percent of the fiber we eat is insoluble and passes through the body and out in the stool (it absorbs water and adds bulk to your stool, which helps with constipation). So one train of thought is that grams of carbs from fiber shouldn't count because they aren't broken down by the body anyhow. But because 20 to 25 percent of fiber grams are soluble, the body breaks down and digests a small percentage of those carbs in the colon (about 1-2 calories per gram of soluble fiber). Your weight loss could stall if those grams are not counted. Many obesity medicine specialists (myself included), recommend counting *total* carbs.

Be sure to eat an abundance of leafy green vegetables to avoid constipation. Leafy green vegetables, such as spinach, lettuce, cabbage, and collards, are a natural way to keep the bowels working regularly. Such greens are rich in fiber, which helps to cleanse the digestive tract. But if you happen to experience the discomfort of constipation, try Colace (docusate) or Metamucil (psyllium), stool softeners that can get the bowels moving again. If you still do not get relief, use Milk of Magnesia, an old, reliable remedy that also helps to replenish the body's magnesium. Take it at bedtime, and by morning, you should be able to take reading materials with you into the bathroom. Drinking lots of water (8 to 10 glasses per day) also helps avoid constipation. If you are not fond of water, try a sparkling version, or if you tend to forget to drink it, buy a large, insulated water bottle and keep the water nice and cold on your desk so you can sip all day.

Don't worry if you experience symptoms; it's called the "keto flu." First of all, I hate the term "keto flu." It sounds far too serious, like you've got a deadly disease. But relax, it's not even a real flu, the symptoms are short-lived, and not everybody experiences them. It's called a "flu" because the symptoms that some people experience while making the transition to a low-carb lifestyle mimic the flu. This happens most frequently if you are eating fewer than 50 carbs a day, and the body goes into the fat-burning ketosis state. Many of my patients don't experience these symptoms because their carb number is above 50, and they don't have to experience a significant ketosis to start losing weight. But for some of you, the symptoms may include headache, fatigue, dizziness, nausea, lethargy, difficulty concentrating or falling asleep, and more. Your blood pressure may even drop, but don't get alarmed. Many of these symptoms occur because a low-carb diet is effective at getting rid of excess water, which can cause dehydration.

As discussed, the purpose of limiting carbs in the diet is to push the body to burn fat for fuel. When that occurs, the fat breaks down into organic compounds, acids called ketones, which can be defined as the energy used in the fat-burning process. But ketones also act as a diuretic, essentially flushing urine from your kidneys. In addition, lowering your insulin level also causes you to excrete urine. So, the resulting symptoms are more like keto dehydration (I prefer that term!). But you can quickly feel better by replacing the salt and water you are losing. I recommend you drink two cups of bouillon soup per day if you develop these symptoms. Each cup provides 500 to 1,000 mg of salt and can provide a quick boost of energy. You can also try bone broth, made by simmering meat bones, which also is a popular treatment for keto flu. You can find many recipes for the broth online.

Be mindful that foods sometimes contain hidden carbs. If you are following the program faithfully, and your weight loss suddenly stalls, the problem may be hidden carbs. The way the food is prepared, especially in restaurants, may affect its carb content. Those factors are difficult to identify if you don't prepare the food yourself. For example, scrambled eggs contain less than one gram of carbs under normal circumstances, but to my amazement, I learned that one restaurant chain cooks its scrambled eggs in pancake batter. That, of course, will affect the carb content of the eggs. And restaurants are notorious for adding sugar in unexpected dishes. This is why I recommend staying at least 5 to 10 carb grams below your number. This helps to compensate for the unknown. More and more restaurants post their nutrition information online or provide it in pamphlet form. Don't be shy about asking for it, and you can always check the restaurant's website. Also, your food tracking app has nutritional information for many of the big food chains, so the information is indeed out there. Of note, legislation from the Affordable Care Act of 2010 now requires certain chain restaurants to have the nutritional information available for all their food.

Try To Get 100 Grams Of Protein Per Day. You may wonder how much protein you should be eating. I purposely haven't talked about this much because first I wanted to focus on getting your carbs right. But protein is just as important. It helps maintain your muscle mass. For starters, most people should shoot for a protein goal of 100 grams per day. Try your best to get your protein from food; that will help to control your hunger and cravings (remember the Hunger Gremlin?). But if you find it difficult to eat that much protein, drink one to two low-carb protein shakes to get to a goal of 100 grams per day. There are a number of these kinds of shakes on the market. Read the label! It should have 20-30 grams or more of protein and less than 10 grams of carbs. Some popular brands are Premier and Muscle Milk, but there are many others. If you have medical issues (like kidney issues), your doctor may want you to limit your protein, so again, make sure you consult your health care provider before starting this or any weight management program.

Now you know all there is to know about Phase One of the No Guesswork Plan. You are on your way to a healthier, happier you! You can pause here to get Phase One solidly in gear before you move on to the rest of the book. Or, you may choose to keep reading to get a preview of what's ahead. If you find yourself struggling to stay committed to a low-carb lifestyle in this high-carb world, read the next two chapters. Either way, there is no reason for delay. Get started with Phase One now!

Just one more thing: When you are four weeks into the NGW Plan, please come back here and take just a few moments to answer seven questions from the Hunt Motivational Scale (HMS) on the following page (go to www.noguesswork to print and fill out the form). If your weight loss stalls as you go through the program, we will ask you to answer them again. The HMS predicts how well you will do on this plan based on how well you scored. If your score is low, focus on improving the areas where you scored low and your weight loss will pick up again.

Also, once you've finished Phase One by losing 10 percent of your starting weight, fill in your name and date on the Award Certificate at the end of this chapter. In addition, please look for the NGW group on Facebook and follow us on social media, join our community of supporters, and post before and after photos at this point so you can be recognized. Also, feel free to share your delicious recipes and the low-carb tips you find.

This is an important milestone on your health journey. You deserve a big pat on the back!

HUNT MOTIVATIONAL SCALE
ACTIVE WEIGHT LOSS (PHASE 1 &2)

PATIENT NAME: ______________________________________

Date:________________

IN THE PAST 2 WEEKS, HOW WELL HAVE YOU DONE THE FOLLOWING:

1. Tracks Food:

0 (rarely)	1 (inconsistently)	2 (consistently)
0-3 days/week	4-5 days/week	>5 days/week

2. Tracks Steps:

0 (never)	1 (inconsistently)	2 (consistently)
0-3 days/week	4-5 days/week	>5 days/week

3. Meals eaten at home meet your carb (or calorie) goal:

0 (never)	1 (inconsistently)	2 (consistently)
0-3 days/week	4-5 days/week	>5 days/week

4. Of the times that you snack, made low-carb choices:
(If person doesn't snack, circle 2.)

0 (never)	1 (inconsistently)	2 (consistently)
<50% of the time	50-80% of the time	More than 80% of the time

5. How many times have you gone out* to eat? Of those times, how often did you plan and then execute a low-carb (or low-calorie) strategy:
(If person hasn't gone out to eat, circle 2.)

0 (never)	1 (inconsistently)	2 (consistently)
<50% of the time	50-80% of the time	More than 80% of the time

*vacation is considered eating out

6. Reach your physical activity (NEAT* + exercise) goals that you and the provider have agreed upon:

0 (rarely)	1 (inconsistently)	2 (consistently)
<50% of the time	50-80% of the time	More than 80% of the time

*NEAT = non exercise activity thermogenesis

7. Reach your carbohydrate (or caloric) goal of X for the day:
   - 0 (not avoiding obvious carbs or calories or getting to goal 3 days or less out of the week)
   - 1 (inconsistently avoiding obvious carbs or calories (getting to goal 4-5 days of the wk). May or may not be tracking)
   - 4 (consistently avoiding obvious carbs or calories (getting to goal more than 5 days/wk). Has to be tracking)

Score: __________

11-16 (predicts that you will do well)

7-10 (Average score. Predicts you may or may not do well in the program. Work to get your number in the 11-16 range)

4-6 (Below average. Predicts you may not do well in the program. Work to get number in the 11-16 range)

0-3 (Predicts you likely will not do well in this program. Do (or redo) an online readiness questionnaire and reassess if this is the right time for you to do a program such as this)

inconsistently means: (1) tracks inconsistently (i.e. 4-5 days of the wk) or (2) doesn't track at all, just tries to avoid obvious carbs/calories (i.e. estimating them in your head) or (3) a little of both

consistently is defined as 80%-100% of the time (more than 5 days of the week)

NGW

NO GUESSWORK CERTIFICATE OF ACHIEVEMENT

IS AWARDED TO

____

For Completion of Phase 1

Weight Management Program

RAMECK HUNT

RAMECK HUNT, MD, FACP

CHAPTER 6

The Keto Question

Is the No Guesswork Plan a keto diet? That's one of the questions people ask most frequently about my program. The short answer is no. No Guesswork is a low-carb program, but not necessarily a ketogenic one. However, the personalized carb numbers for some people on the plan may be low enough to fall within the range of a ketogenic diet. Others on my plan may *choose* to forgo their higher personalized carb numbers and keep their carbs in the low keto range to lose weight faster. And guess what? That's fine! Why? A ketogenic diet is perfectly healthy, safe, and sustainable.

I know that goes against what *they* (the keto critics) say. I'll address that in a moment. But first, let's recap the difference between a low-carb diet and a ketogenic diet. In my opinion, there is no significant difference between the two in terms of what happens to the body to cause you to lose weight. The difference is in the numbers. A low-carb diet by definition is the consumption of 50 to 150 grams of carbs per day. A ketogenic diet caps the number of carb grams at 50 per day (or less than 20 grams of NET carbs, which is the carb grams minus the grams of fiber). So, if your personalized carb number under No Guesswork is, say, 60, 75, or 90, you technically aren't following a ketogenic diet. But if your No Guesswork carb number is 50, 40, or 25, your diet is considered keto. Nevertheless, if you're losing weight, the same physiology is happening on the inside of you with either plan. You are burning fat instead of carbs and producing ketones for fuel. A similar process happens to all of us overnight when we "fast" while we are sleeping. Our bodies use ketones overnight for fuel. Ketones are essential for survival. There are so many good things about ketones, one of which is that they are satiating. So when you burn fat you produce ketones and those ketones make you less hungry.

So, once again, the keto diet is a healthy one. Not everyone thinks so, however. With the rise in popularity of keto, the critics' voices are rising, too. They've rendered keto guilty of a host of untrue claims, but let's cross-examine what *they* say, and you be the judge.

Safety of the Keto Diet

"A keto diet isn't safe." That's the main criticism you will hear. My question is, says who? If you ask those who believe this nonsense why, you get strange answers or a blank stare. FACT: Medical doctors prescribe ketogenic diets for children to treat intractable seizures. This is well documented. It is SAFE and very effective. Now, follow the logic. If a ketogenic diet is safe enough for children, why wouldn't it be safe for adults? In fact, we doctors also recommend a ketogenic diet for adults who suffer from intractable seizures.

"A keto diet makes you lose water weight." Um, okay, and the problem is what? That's what popped into my head when I heard this one at a medical conference I attended for internal medicine. More than 50,000 physicians from all over the world regularly attend this conference, so the presenters have much influence in the profession. I sat there, a bit in shock as I heard this comment mentioned casually during one session, as if there's something wrong with losing water weight. FACT: in many cases, losing water weight is a very good thing. It's true that some people may lose water weight and experience keto dehydration (or what some people call "the keto flu," a term I detest) in the first few weeks while their bodies adapt to the keto lifestyle. But, as I've mentioned, rehydration is an easy fix. You can make sure you have enough salt in your diet by consuming bone broth or bouillon. It's also important to get enough potassium and magnesium (primarily via foods or supplements) because your body may be depleted of these in the beginning, as well. The truth is that losing extra water weight with a keto diet can significantly decrease the swelling in your legs (edema). I have many patients who had to take water pills to control the water weight in their legs. And many of them were able to get off their

water pills with a low-carb or keto diet because these diets got rid of their excess water weight.

"A keto diet depletes you of essential vitamins and minerals." This boils down to individual choices. If you choose a well-formulated keto diet, you won't be depleted of any vitamins or minerals. Meat and fish are loaded with vitamins and minerals, and so is the yolk of an egg. They are all also important protein sources. Some research has shown that a keto diet may deprive the body of one or two micronutrients, such as manganese. But any diet that is not well-formulated can leave you depleted of needed nutrients. My answer to that is to take a multivitamin, just to be sure you are getting all of the nutrients you need to stay healthy.

"A keto diet doesn't have carbs and you need carbs for survival and health." That's the lie we've all been fed. We discussed in an earlier chapter how this happened. The medical truth is you don't need to eat carbs to survive. In fact the opposite is true; you need ketones to survive (when you sleep your body has to be fueled by ketones in order for you to survive). The body does need about 110 to 140 grams of carbs (i.e. glucose) to fuel your brain, but your system makes enough of these carbs on its own to do the job (about twice as much). In fact, a man's body makes about 250 grams of carbs per day via a process called gluconeogenesis and glycogenolysis. Furthermore, your brain can use ketones for about 80 percent of the energy that it needs (remember ketones are essential for life). So that means you need only about 25 to 30 grams of actual carbs to fuel your brain, and your body makes eight times that amount on its own (gluconeogenesis/glycogenolysis). This information comes from the Institute of Medicine (IOM), which gives us researched recommendations on the intake requirements for nutrients (among many other recommendations). The IOM is made up of scientists and other eminent professionals who advise the federal government on matters of medical care, research, and education, and they have said that we don't need to eat carbs for survival or health. In fact, of the three macronutrients (proteins, carbohydrates, and fats), only one is non-essential: carbohydrates. There are nine essential proteins (amino acids) and two essential fats that we have to consume for health and survival.

"A keto diet is bad for your cholesterol." We talked about this at length in Chapter Two (The Fat Truth), but let's recap this point here. First, we have to break down what cholesterol is. Briefly, cholesterol is made by all animal cells and is an essential structural component for all your cell membranes. Cholesterol is also essential for making steroid hormones (testosterone, estrogen, etc.) in the human body. So we need cholesterol for life. We also eat foods that have cholesterol in them. And most of the cholesterol that we ingest is esterified. Esterified cholesterol can't be absorbed, so most of it passes through and comes out in the stool. Our body also recycles cholesterol in the un-esterified form bile (the absorbable form). The absorption of the small percentage of un-esterified cholesterol that is in the foods we eat has to compete with the reabsorption of the un-esterified cholesterol your body excretes. Because of this, only a small portion of the cholesterol you eat actually gets absorbed. To demonstrate this point, there is an FDA approved medication (Zetia) that prevents the absorption of cholesterol from your gut, which decreases your cholesterol by about 15 percent, about the amount that dietary cholesterol affects the cholesterol in your body.

Cholesterol and triglycerides are transported through your blood via proteins (lipoproteins). These proteins are either good (HDL) or bad (LDL). The good cholesterol (HDL) removes fat from the cell wall and decreases atherosclerosis, the cause of heart attacks. Think of HDL as a garbage truck; the more garbage trucks (HDL) you have, the cleaner the streets (i.e. your arteries) are. The fewer garbage trucks (HDL) you have, the more garbage (LDL) piles up and blocks the streets (i.e. your arteries).

That's the main thing about your cholesterol. And then there are triglycerides, the fat part. They are categorized into either saturated fats or unsaturated fats. As mentioned in Chapter Two, there is no significant evidence that consumption of saturated fats increases risk of heart disease. However, in general, increased triglycerides have been associated with increased risk of heart disease. Interestingly, decreasing triglycerides with medication doesn't decrease the risk of heart disease. It's my opinion that this is because you are decreasing triglycerides in isolation. The reason that the triglycerides are increased in the first place wasn't addressed: insulin resistance. And as I mentioned, insulin resistance and diabetes are what cause atherosclerosis/coronary artery disease. By not addressing insulin resistance and only decreasing triglycerides, there's no wonder why atherosclerosis and coronary artery disease are not affected.

So now let's answer the question, does a keto diet raise your cholesterol? The short answer is no. It is well documented that a low-carb ketogenic diet raises your good cholesterol (HDL) and lowers your triglycerides (saturated and unsaturated fats), which reduce your risk of heart attacks. So then why do people say a ketogenic diet is bad for your cholesterol? A part of it is because a ketogenic diet can sometimes increase your bad cholesterol (LDL); sometimes, however, it stays the same. But overall your good cholesterol (HDL) goes up, your triglycerides go down, and your bad cholesterol (LDL) may go up or stay the same. So when you add it up, your cholesterol, overall, gets better, not worse. Anecdotally, every aspect of my cholesterol got much better on a ketogenic diet: HDL, triglycerides and, yes, even my LDL.

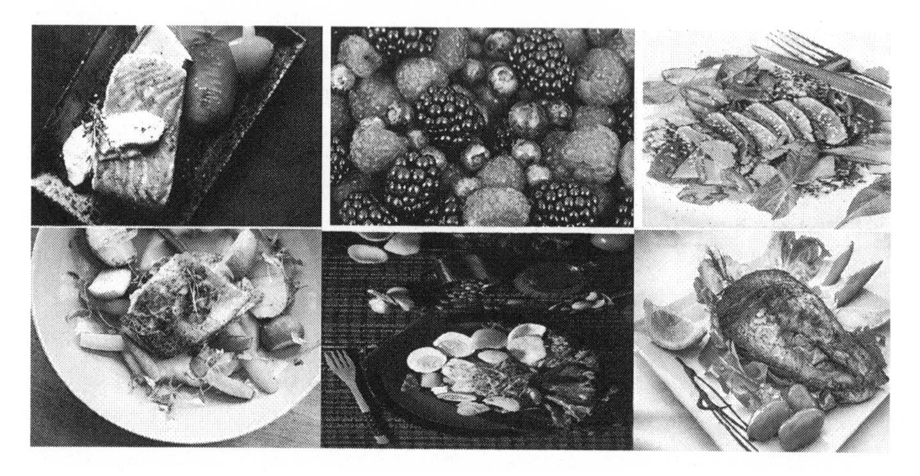

Why does bad cholesterol (LDL) go up for some people when they're on a keto diet? Well, all ketogenic diets are not well formulated. Just like all vegetarian diets are not necessarily good. I have many vegetarian patients who have uncontrolled diabetes because they are eating a lot sugars and refined carbohydrates (bread, sweets, pasta, potatoes, etc.,). The same with a ketogenic diet. If you are always eating charred meat, processed meat, your HDL will still go up and your fats (triglycerides) will go down, but usually your bad cholesterol will go up. But if you are eating a well-formulated low-carb diet, similar to a low-carb Mediterranean diet that's full of fatty fish, like salmon, and salads, and green leafy vegetables and avocados, your cholesterol will likely be the best you've ever had.

There are many people out there who live a low-carb lifestyle and are healthy and happy, including myself. So the next time people say this to you (a keto diet is bad for your health), tell them they are stupid liars (okay, maybe you shouldn't say that exactly, but thinking it won't hurt). And refer them to the IOM report.

Keto Diet Studies

"A keto diet doesn't have long-term studies to prove that it's safe." That's simply not true. There are prospective randomized long-term (greater than a year) studies of ketogenic diets that have been completed, and there are more underway. (A prospective randomized trial is the gold standard of the way to do research. It follows people going forward (not in the past) in real time and those people are randomly picked to be a part of one group or the other group being tested, in an effort not to have any bias.)

But what about the adults who have been doing a keto diet for thirty years to control their seizures ever since they were little kids? Is the study of them not long-term enough? This is a pet peeve of mine. Just because ketogenic diets don't yet have randomized prospective studies that have lasted five, ten, or twenty years doesn't mean that they should be assumed to be unsafe. That's not logical thinking, especially when we have many retrospective, very long-term studies (with twenty to thirty years of follow-up) that say keto diets — used for controlling seizures — are very safe and effective. And there are many shorter-term prospective studies that demonstrate how safe a keto diet is and how it improves your metabolic parameters (such as insulin resistance, diabetes, good HDL cholesterol and triglycerides, blood pressure, inflammation, etc.)

Why would anyone just assume a keto diet is unsafe when there is no good evidence of that? Most of the available evidence shows the opposite, that a keto diet is safe and healthy in terms of blood markers for the heart. Unfortunately, many have deemed keto guilty until proven innocent. That's not the way justice (or science) is supposed to operate, right? The ironic part is that there are studies on America's favorite diet, the low-fat diet (by definition a high-carb diet), and although there are some studies that show benefit, many have shown that cardiovascular risk factors, like cholesterol, sugar, inflammatory markers, etc., are worse under a low-fat diet than a low-carb diet. And some studies even showed that people on high-carb diets have increased mortality than people in a high-fat group. In fact, one such study, the Look Ahead trial, which was supposed to evaluate whether a low-fat diet would improve heart health for people with type 2 diabetes, had to be stopped early because those conducting the study believed it would have been unethical to continue it. So even though there are studies that show the overall ineffectiveness of low-fat diets, many people and organizations still recommend them.

Let's get this straight. We know a low-fat diet has been shown not to be helpful in some studies and may be harmful based on some short-term, long-term, and very long-term studies. And we know that a keto diet may be helpful based on short-term and long-term studies, but because there are no *very* long-term studies, some have claimed arbitrarily that it is not safe. And instead, they recommend a low-fat diet? In many cases, yes, medical experts from influential organizations still recommend low-fat diets. Look it up. Basically all I am saying here is, they should be measured by the same stick, and they are not.

FACT: The multi-million-dollar Look AHEAD study, funded by taxpayer dollars, didn't show any benefit of a low-fat diet on heart health. It had to be stopped early because of its overall futility.

FACT: Another trial, called the WHI study, also funded by taxpayer dollars, showed that a low-fat diet did not benefit your heart, prevent you from having a stroke, or help reduce invasive breast cancer.

FACT: Yet another multi-million-dollar study, known as the Nurses Study (yes, funded by taxpayer dollars), showed that a low-fat diet did not reduce breast cancer.

Question: When will taxpayer dollars be spent on studying the low-carb diet to determine its long-term safety and effectiveness, instead of continuing to spend taxpayer money on the low-fat diet, which has failed time and time again?

Innocent Until Proven Guilty

Most of the evidence available thus far points to the safety and effectiveness of a keto diet. So my position is *innocent until proven guilty*, not the other way around. I'm not sure why some of my fellow doctor colleagues spin it the other way, given that they *should* know the facts. Sure, we have to continue to consider longer term data when it is available, but from what we know now and from my own long-term experience with my patients (and myself), a keto diet is safe and effective in the long term. And yet, there are even more criticisms.

"There is entirely too much fat in a keto diet!" Again, I ask, what's wrong with that? As I explained earlier, when compared to sugar and refined carbs (I'm not talking about fiber here), fat is healthier. Having high sugar in your blood (i.e. diabetes/pre-diabetes/insulin resistance) puts you at risk for heart attacks and strokes, even if you have lower cholesterol. This is why doctors have to lower the cholesterol of diabetics, even lower than recommended for the general population, to make sure the high sugar doesn't cause a heart attack or stroke. So, sugar and refined carbohydrates put you at greater risk for heart disease and strokes than a diet high in fat. Remember the Maasai from Africa? Also, what diet has been proven to be the best for heart health? A high fat diet — the Mediterranean Diet. The PREDIMED study, that proved this, recommended a diet that was more than 60 percent fat. Case closed.

Allow me to clarify something. I said that I do keto. But I don't purposely try to do keto. It has become a lifestyle, and I just stay away from sugars and refined carbohydrates. That means I end up being in the keto range most days, but not every day. Still, I stay below my carb maintenance number for sure, almost always.

I view sugar and refined carbohydrates like most people view fat. When I see sugar (cookies, cakes, pies, etc.) and refined carbs (potatoes, French fries, bread, etc.), I think: "THAT'S A HEART ATTACK WAITING TO HAPPEN!" This is the same way a person with diabetes (or pre-diabetes and insulin resistance) should look at food that would make the sugar in their blood go up and puts them at risk for a heart attack or stroke. Sugar and refined carbs are to your arteries like acid is to a pipe. And carbs can fuel cancer. So, I just stay away from them, the same way that many people avoid fat. Actually, we all would be healthier if we looked at carbs that way. Take that same energy you applied to stay away from fat and transfer it to avoid carbs.

Tell The Truth

What I say to my colleagues is simple: report the facts. Don't continue to demonize a keto diet by saying it's all processed meats, full of bacon, salami, burgers, etc. As I mentioned, a well-formulated ketogenic diet is a colorful diet, full of avocados, nuts, grass-fed meats, oily fish, etc. Ultimately, the diet I recommend, based on available evidence, is a low-carb Mediterranean diet in the Maintenance Phase, which, if you are up to it, you can start implementing at any phase of the program. The sooner the better.

This might stir up the big companies that have profited from the low-fat lies. But when will my profession as a whole stop hanging onto these old beliefs that have been shown to be untrue (fat is bad and sugar and refined carbs are okay)? When will we care enough about people to tell the whole truth? That is what I seek to do with this book, even if it means I have to take some heat. And I'm not saying processed foods are good for you, because they are not. There are several studies which clearly show that they are not and can be harmful in the long term. So, I do not recommend consuming processed foods like bacon in abundance over time. But a little bacon once in a while is fine, particularly in the beginning. I am also not saying there aren't other diets out there that are good for people. For example, a well-formulated, plant-based diet is a very good diet, based on the studies. But does it check off all the boxes for my 6 S's (Simple, Safe, Sustainable, Satisfying, Superior (for weight loss than other diets), and Sugarless)? You may not be able to Sustain a plant-based diet as long as a low-carb diet (though some may), and you may not be able to achieve as much weight loss as you would by avoiding carbs. For the majority of people, staying away from carbs and refined carbohydrates is the safest bet. And that's what my No Guesswork Plan helps you to do.

Are all low-carb diets good for you? Not if they're not well-formulated. Just as with an unhealthy vegetarian diet, you can have an unhealthy low-carb diet, full of processed meat, charred meat, and a paucity of vegetables. But that's not what my low-carb diet is. My No Guesswork low-carb diet is full of healthy fats, fiber, and protein.

One more note before we leave this subject. Let's be clear: Research studies are a "testing environment." People who sign up to participate, particularly for nutrition studies, are motivated enough to be part of the research. Their behavior may be different than others who did not bother to participate. Nutrition studies are largely based on behaviors and behavior modification. So, research cannot tell us *exactly* what would happen in the real world. But it's the best we can do, ethically.

Look, nutritional science doesn't have all the answers. But we do know a low-fat diet has not served the population well over the last fifty years. We have been experimenting with it in the real world for so long and look where it has gotten us, nowhere. We as a whole have not lost weight; in fact, we are gaining weight at alarming rates. The prevalence of diabetes and heart disease is increasing, not decreasing, as proponents of the low-fat diet predicted. And fat had nothing to do with these alarming increases (because our fat percentage decreased); sugar and refined carbs increased and are mostly to blame. Yes, we should move more, and yes, we should decrease our portions (among other things, like smoking, etc.). But the main culprits when we're talking about obesity, diabetes, and heart disease, are sugar and refined carbs. And if we can significantly reduce those through a low-carb diet and a ketogenic diet, we can begin to see an improvement in health for us all.

Is that NGW-APPROVED?

So I ask you: Is what you're eating NGW-APPROVED? If not, I urge you to get in on this NGW lifestyle and ride the NGW wave.

CHAPTER 7

Thriving in a High-Carb World

You're excited, motivated, and ready to win the weight loss battle on the No Guesswork Plan. Then, a few days in — maybe you forget your lunch at home, or get invited to a party after work, or just show up at work as usual on Donut Day — and reality hits you. Carbs are everywhere. Carbs you used to *love* are everywhere. And the low-carb options? Not so much. And you start to wonder: *Can I succeed on this plan when I'm constantly bombarded with carbs? Can I live without carbs forever? Is a low-carb lifestyle really sustainable over the long haul?*

The short answer is *absolutely*! I know firsthand because I've maintained this lifestyle for several years, and I'm healthier and happier than I've ever been. And keep in mind, I thought I'd *never* learn to live without pizza (seems like that's all we ate in medical school). I didn't take some magic pill to fall out of love with pizza. But I came to realize that to make my new lifestyle permanent, I had to change my mindset. That means I decided I could no longer do the same things the same way. So the response is not difficult now when people ask me in astonishment, "You haven't eaten pizza in five or six years?" I just shrug it off and say, "No, I don't eat pizza." (Quite honestly, pizza doesn't even taste as amazing as I once remembered. In fact, many people's taste changes over time once they haven't had something in a while, as did mine; it's like when you reduce your salt intake, and after a while, foods that you once loved taste too salty). Sometimes, I fill in the blank with whatever happens to be the source of their amazement—bread, rice, pasta, or sweets. I just don't think about those things because I know they are unhealthy and can lead to obesity. I don't want to be unhealthy or have obesity, so I don't indulge. That doesn't mean I've never eaten *any* high-carb foods since I started this lifestyle. It's just such a rare occurrence, and I don't feel deprived because I don't focus on what I no longer want or what I can't have. And if I can do it, you can, too. Throughout this book, you will meet some of my patients who got down to their goal weight on the NGW plan and have maintained that weight loss for years.

Among the patients whose success has impressed me the most is an awesome twenty-seven-year-old man with autism, whom I will call Dominick. I met him in the summer of 2019, after I began offering my weight management program at the hospital clinic for patients who are uninsured or covered by Medicaid. I was eager to reach this vulnerable population of patients because they often don't get this kind of comprehensive care. Dominick came in with his mother, who is his primary caretaker, to be treated for a sinus infection. But while providing his medical information, the mother mentioned that her son needed to lose about thirty pounds. He had begun anti-psychotic medication to stabilize his mood, but the drug had caused tremendous weight gain. An avid swimmer, Dominick had become sluggish and was beginning to complain of joint pains. He also was pre-diabetic and had little energy to participate in the day program he had once enjoyed.

Initially, Dominick appeared withdrawn when I tried to interact with him. He stared down at the floor and gave one-word answers. His mother answered the questions I asked him. But I sensed there was something special about Dominick. While he played around on his mobile phone, his mother told me how she desperately needed guidance to help Dominick get to a healthier weight. He had gained thirty to forty pounds in just a year after beginning the medication. I had the perfect plan for him, I told Dominick's mother, before describing NGW. She was initially reluctant. How would a patient with autism who also has mild Obsessive Compulsive Disorder be able to follow such a regimen? I told her that we would make One Simple Consistent Change (remember OSCC?) at a time, and she agreed to start the journey.

We began by focusing on keeping Dominick's carb intake to under 100 grams per day (with a target of 75 grams/day), and to make that happen we swapped out a few items in his diet. We substituted berries for his usual banana at breakfast, and veggie omelets for his oatmeal. Since I'd noticed that Dominick was somewhat of a techie, I encouraged him to begin tracking his carbs. That kind of engagement for Dominick proved to be extremely useful. He loved tracking; it was, to him, a game. When he returned in five weeks, he'd lost three pounds. His mother wasn't blown away, but I reminded her that our journey was a marathon, not a sprint. We found his carb number to be 80, and carefully implemented a few more changes (such as veggies and dip for a snack instead of cookies), and Dominick kept swimming three times a week. His mother had to be careful when making changes to his routine because the slightest difference might leave him agitated. At his next visit, I shared with Dominick the good news: "You lost another three pounds!"

His response was enthusiastic: "Yes, I did! I did!"

Dominick was thrilled to show off his meticulous tracking, and over time, he continued warming up to me. When he weighed in for the fourth time, he'd lost seven pounds for that visit alone, and his mother had become a believer. For each subsequent visit, his weight kept going down—he lost one pound, then five pounds, then four pounds, and more. By the seventh month, Dominick was down from 230 pounds to 203. He had lost nearly thirty pounds, which was his goal. Thrilled with his progress, his mom admitted that she had set the goal conservatively at thirty pounds, with little expectation that he would be able to achieve it. "Can we keep going?" she asked, as a smile spread across her usually stern face.

Dominick's journey continues, but he is no longer pre-diabetic, and every one of his health markers has improved. I am confident that Dominick, with his mother's help, will be able to sustain his success.

*****

Now, there is more than just anecdotal evidence about the long-term success and sustainability of a low-carb lifestyle. A three-year observational study, published in January 2014, concluded that a moderate low-carbohydrate diet (defined as between 70 and 130 grams of carbs per day) was "highly effective, safe, and sustainable." As part of that study, researchers followed 200 Japanese patients with Type II diabetes for over three years. The patients were instructed to follow a moderate low-carb meal plan (70-130 grams of carbs per day), while various health indicators, including body weight and blood sugar levels for diabetes, were tracked. The study showed that not only did the vast majority of the patients sustain the lifestyle, but their health in several different areas improved, as well.

So, let's put this question of sustainability to rest. You *can* lose weight, and you *can* keep it off for the rest of your life on my low-carb plan. Let your personalized carb number be your guide; if you stick to that limit, you'll know how many carbs you can eat and still lose weight. But staying true to the low-carb lifestyle requires two additional important things, perhaps more than anything else: You must commit to it, and you also must plan to succeed. It really is as simple as that.

Commitment requires discipline and dedication. But sometimes, just as in relationships, people fear the commitment because they are so focused on what they must give up. When I first met one of my patients, Lori, a technology consultant in her mid-40s, she made a firm pronouncement as soon as we sat down to talk: "Look, I can't give up carbs!" Married to a doctor, Lori had heard about my plan and come to me somewhat reluctantly upon his recommendation, after telling him repeatedly that she wanted to lose weight and get healthier. She was experiencing bad knee pain and other joint ailments, but she wanted to let me know from the start that this low-carb thing just wasn't for her. "I travel. I eat on the go," she added. "I'm not going to be able to do this."

I listened patiently and told Lori that she could surely try a low-calorie approach if she insisted but that science has shown a low-carb approach to be better for weight loss, as well as healthier. I explained the insulin response that is triggered inside the body by a high-carb, low-calorie diet and told her that if she changed her focus, she would be amazed by all she *could* eat. I suggested some alternatives, like eating her burgers in a lettuce wrap or with a knife and fork or ordering grilled chicken nuggets or tenders, instead of the battered ones. And I made a deal with her: if she tried the low-carb approach for just two weeks and found it completely unmanageable, we would try something different.

When Lori returned for her checkup, she had lost five pounds. She was shocked and ecstatic. "You know, it wasn't as bad as I thought it was going to be," she said.

She lost 35 pounds over a period of 16 weeks, and the change in her diet reduced the inflammation in her joints. The knee pain that she had been experiencing went away, which helped to keep her motivated to stay on the plan.

When my patients complain that they can't give up carbs, I often ask, "What if I told you that you have diabetes or that you are lactose intolerant?" Think about that for a moment. As upsetting as that would be, I'm willing to bet most people would start to think of how to eat in a whole new way, and they would be willing to make the dietary sacrifices for the sake of their health. Well, committing to a low-carb lifestyle is no less important. I suggest thinking of yourself as "carb-intolerant." Just like those who are lactose intolerant give up foods they previously enjoyed (even ice cream!) because of the destruction those foods cause to their bodies, you may have to think of pasta, breads, and sweets in the same way. Telling people that you are "carb intolerant" may make them laugh, but it's a gracious way to decline food from that person who always insists that you eat some of her potato salad or sweet potato pie.

Again, instead of focusing on the foods you have to exclude from your diet, think of this as an exciting time of exploration. You can try new vegetables that you've never eaten before and experiment with new ways of cooking them. You can discover new recipes and find substitutes for your old, unhealthy staples. But most of all, you can eat until you're satisfied.

Even in this high-carb world, you can thrive with a low-carb lifestyle. How? Well, here are a few tips that can help you adjust, until the low-carb life and my NGW plan become just part of who you are.

Equip Your Home For Success

Your home is your first line of defense against failure. So set it up for success. If possible, carb-proof your environment. Get rid of all of the sugary, starchy carbs you won't be eating! Who wants your space filled with tempting carbs that you can't eat? That would be a bit like keeping your ex-lovers around after you've moved on. You especially don't want them hanging around when you've had a bad or stressful day. They're not good for you; you know they're not good for you. But when you're tired, frustrated, or not thinking straight, you're much more likely to indulge. Then comes the guilt. So save yourself the trouble. Clean out those pantries!

Of course, carb-proofing your home is easier to do if you live alone. If you share your space with a spouse, children, or other family members or friends who are not committed to low-carb living, they might not appreciate your cleaning spree. I'm not suggesting you start a civil war in your home. It's okay to be considerate. You just may have to rearrange some things to create a space in the refrigerator and the pantry for your stuff. Then, make a trip to the grocery (or place an order online) and fill your spaces with the foods you can enjoy — an array of meats, poultry, seafood, non-starchy vegetables (fresh and frozen), avocados, eggs, cheeses, berries, nuts, and more.

You are much more likely to stay on track if you have on hand foods that can be prepared easily or grabbed quickly when you must eat on the run. It's easy to fall back into the old way of preparing food and eating when you are pressed for time and can't put your hands on low-carb foods or snacks. And these days, who isn't pressed for time? So, stay prepared!

Plan Your Meals

You will hear me say again and again that planning is key to success on the NGW plan. Your meal plan is your game plan. Without it, you are making up the plays as you go. You might get lucky and win the game that way, but you are much more likely to reach your goal if you plan to win. Come up with a meal-by-meal plan for each day, including snacks, and stick to it. When you know exactly what you're going to eat, you can avoid the temptations on your favorite take-out menus at mealtime. It's okay if your plan includes a take-out meal, but if you're stopping at the place to order, know ahead of time what you plan to get (and its carb content) so that you don't have to spend time studying the menu on the spot. It's always more difficult to resist the tantalizing photos of decadent, carb-rich foods when you're uncertain and hungry. So, look up the menu online ahead of time. Most restaurants now make their menus available on their websites. Your game plan tells you exactly what to do, so there's little time to veer off course.

Many people go beyond just planning to meal prepping, preparing full meals for the week — or at least, doing the tedious steps, such as dicing veggies or slicing meats — in advance. The meals are appropriately portioned and stored in the refrigerator or freezer in plastic containers, baggies, or glass jars until it's time to warm or cook. There's really no right or wrong way to meal prep, but you can find lots of detailed suggestions and best practices on the internet. The point is to find a strategy that works for you, whether it's preparing a week's worth of fully-cooked, individual meals that can be microwaved at lunch or assembling family-sized portions that can go from the fridge to the dinner table for your entire crew with just one additional step.

Ellie, a patient of mine in her thirties who works as a busy office manager, likes to meal prep on Sundays. She and her partner set aside a portion of each Sunday to prepare each meal for the entire week. They store the meals individually in plastic containers, put some in the refrigerator and some in the freezer, and then take them out to reheat, as needed. That simple step helped Ellie lose 25 pounds without feeling like she was on a diet.

I recommend picking a day that works for you. Then prep your meals for the work week (Monday through Friday). To keep meal planning simple and quick, you also might consider giving certain days of the week a meal theme, such as Taco Tuesdays (with your favorite lettuce replacing the taco shell, of course), Friday Fish, or Soul Food Sundays. At least on those days, you won't have to spend much time thinking about what to prepare for dinner.

Be Mindful of Breakfast

The WORST meal of the day, hands down, is breakfast! By worst, I mean the meal most loaded with sugar. For most people, the sugar content of breakfast amounts to eating a bowl filled with sugar, whether it's cereal or a donut, muffin, bagel — you name the carb. If it's a breakfast food, it's most likely full of sugar or refined carbohydrates. Food companies have fed us with the notion that breakfast is the most important meal of the day. But is it really? Studies say, that, too, is just a myth. But for the sake of argument, let's just say breakfast is as important as we've been taught to believe. Should you really be eating donuts, cakes, pop tarts, muffins (all just sugar) for the most important meal of the day? Of course not. Even proponents of a low-fat diet would probably agree with that.

You can eat breakfast, if you like, but cut out the sugary stuff that may be in your pantry. Enjoy a protein—maybe a breakfast meat, such as sausage, bacon, or lox (without the bagel) with some sautéed spinach or a frittata. Or just have a vegetable omelet, scrambled eggs, or hard-boiled eggs for breakfast. If you're on the run, a protein shake also might suffice. And if you're bored with bacon or sausage, who ever said chicken or fish can't be breakfast meats? In some countries, it is customary to eat fish for breakfast. Open up your options and stop making excuses.

Thrive At Work

In just about every workplace, there are the co-workers who bring donuts for the staff to have in the mornings, or home-baked goods (cookies or brownies) to nibble throughout the day. Then there are the office birthday cakes and occasional pot-luck lunches. Those things you can't control. You have to just say no to the sweet, starchy stuff, but doing so is easier when the Hunger Gremlin (your ghrelin level) is low. So stay nourished! This is where planning is important. See, what I do in those situations is I have a little cubbyhole where I have a stash of tasty, low-carb snacks. So, whenever I see them pull out the donuts, I reach for my nuts or cheese sticks, chips (protein chips, of course), or a protein shake and I'm good. The key is to reach for something before your limbic system gets stimulated because at that point it's too late. Once your limbic system starts to spin, you can't stop it by eating protein. You have to do that *before* it starts spinning. There's a scientific term for this: stimulus control (controlling your environment as much as you can by having a plan in place *before* you get tempted). The other term is stimulus narrowing (avoiding temptation by exposing yourself as little as possible to high-carb foods and maintaining your own section of healthy choices in the fridge or pantry).

One of the big advantages of the NGW plan is that you don't have to count calories, which means you can eat heartily (no more semi-starvation or baby meals). You just have to be mindful of how you "spend" your carbs. As I said earlier, think of your carb number as dollars (or cents, as in the example I used in Chapter 5), and every carb in the food you eat represents a dollar that must be subtracted from your total. If you choose foods that have zero or few carbs, your "dollars" can go a long way. Try eating before you leave home in the mornings and keeping a stash of low-carb snacks handy in a desk drawer or file cabinet. This keeps the Hunger Gremlin's growl away. If you feed the beast before it starts to grow, you have a much better chance of being disciplined enough to walk away from the donuts and cake. So, eat smart, and if needed, eat often.

If your workplace has a cafeteria, that's a great convenience and an easy way to fill up on proteins and fats. Of course, there will be plenty high-carb options, but you are strong enough now to skip right over them and look for the delicious chicken/turkey, meat, seafood offerings, non-starchy veggies, and/or a colorful salad. Sometimes, if I'm still hungry between lunch and dinner, I go back to the hospital cafeteria and get a second lunch. I love to eat. Some of my colleagues even think it's funny that the diet/healthy eating guru is so greedy! Of course, I look at it differently. I'm not greedy; I'm just trying to keep my ghrelin low. Thank goodness that's okay under my NGW plan. I just have to be mindful of what I put on my plate. As long as I stick primarily to the proteins and fats, I can go back as often as needed to feel satisfied. This is now a lifestyle for me, as I am hoping it will become for you, as well.

Nowadays, I don't have to think much about food. I know what to eat, I know what I like, and I explore so many low-carb dishes and treats. There are so many more low-carb options out there than I ever knew about. And I like to think about all the things I can have and the things that are good for me, versus what's off limits. If you approach your food like a kid looking in a window, watching all the other kids playing, wishing you could be in there with them, you are setting yourself up for failure. Sooner rather than later, you will go back to eating those things. Instead, think about ALL the things you can have and the new things you want to try.

Dine Out With Confidence

I'm encouraged by the menu options I saw recently in a restaurant. An entire side of the menu was dedicated to paleo options. Paleo is not exactly a low-carb diet, but it is somewhat low in carbs, and that's a sign that more people are recognizing the value of a low-carb lifestyle and demanding more low-carb choices on restaurant menus. So, when you see "paleo" or "low-carb" or "keto" on a menu, those are most likely the options with the fewest amount of carbs. I encourage you to order from that side of the menu. Remember, demand influences the market. If restaurant owners and food companies see a great demand for low-carb foods, they will respond. It's the nature of this beast we call capitalism. That's what happened with the explosion of low-fat foods on the market all those years ago, even without the science to back up the validity of the health claims. Science has again and again shown the health advantages of a low-carb lifestyle, and finally there are signs, like the restaurant menu, that the market is slowly catching up.

Even if your favorite restaurant doesn't offer a special menu, you don't have to fear eating out. Every restaurant that you can imagine has some low-carb choices. Sometimes getting the low-carb meal you desire may be as simple as asking the waiter to substitute the baked potato, rice, or French fries that are often paired with your entrée with green beans, broccoli, or a salad. If your favorite Italian restaurant doesn't offer mashed cauliflower or spiraled zucchini in place of the pasta, just request the meat and sauce with a side of veggies or a salad and account for the sauce in your daily carb allotment. If the family is dining out for barbeque, inquire about getting your chicken or ribs with a dry rub, in place of the barbeque, or try plain smoked. If you are attending a reception or social event with a fixed menu, the choices are more limited, but you still have choices. You can eat beforehand or drink a protein shake so that you feel less tempted to indulge. It's about making good choices, wherever you happen to be dining.

What is the biggest form of entertainment in this country? It's not a concert or TV; it's food! Many of our interactions with family and friends center around food. So, if we restrict or limit what we eat, what do we do for entertainment? The same as before: Eat and enjoy! You just have to make good food choices, and that means no sugary foods or refined carbs. You can do this!

RED LIGHT! GREEN LIGHT!

I might be dating myself, but does anyone remember the game kids used to play, "Red Light, Green Light?" In this game one of the kids playing is chosen to be the "stop light." The rest of the kids, who are about 15 feet away, try to advance in an attempt to touch the kid who is the "stop light." When the kid who is the stop light says "red light!" the other kids have to stop and freeze in place. If the "stop light" kid catches anyone still moving, that kid is out of the game. Whichever kid reaches and touches the "stop light" kid first, wins the game. I was reminded of that game recently when I saw a patient for weight management.

I was talking to one of my patients during a follow-up weigh-in visit and I asked her my usual opening question, "How are you doing with your diet?" And she said something to me that I found interesting and very helpful. "Dr. Hunt, I'm trying to avoid my red light foods." And so I asked her to explain what she meant by "red light foods." And she said "You know, the foods you have to stop at, just like a red light." I thought, wow, that's a great way to look at it. And thinking of it that way I think has been very helpful for my other patients as well. So I incorporate that into my visits when I talk to them about food. And then I added the term "green light foods," foods that you CAN eat, the GO foods, just like a green light, or what we call the NGW-APPROVED foods. This is not a new analogy. Many others use the red light, green light analogy in their own way. Our weight management program is always individualized to you, so we want you to make your own chart, specific for your trigger foods, which are your red light foods. In the same vain we want you to make your own specific chart for the green light GO-TO foods, the NGW-APPROVED foods that you enjoy.

What are some red light foods? We discussed many of them in this book, like potato chips, rice, cake, pasta, etc. So what specifically are your trigger red light foods? I suggest you make a list on paper or a mental list of your red light foods. For example, some of my red light foods used to be chips, pizza, rice, bread. What are yours?

But more importantly, what are your green light foods? The foods that are great for your low-carb lifestyle. Your GO-TO foods that you enjoy. Your NGW-APPROVED foods. My NGW-APPROVED foods are also many of the things we discuss in this book. Things like salmon, turkey, chicken, cheese sticks, and strawberries, among other things. So what are your NGW-APPROVED foods?

Stay Hydrated

I get this question all the time: What should I drink on the NGW plan? You already know the answer, though — it's the same thing your grandmother always told you. Drink plenty of water. Sure, you can have it sparkling, with a twist of lime, lemon, or cucumber. But nothing beats water for quenching a thirst with zero carbs.

In the beginning, you also can drink diet beverages, as long as you add two glasses of water for every one glass (eight ounces) of a diet drink. But keep in mind that there are some studies that suggest artificial sweeteners can impede weight loss. Also, "naturally" sweetened beverages, like the Bai drinks, can be enjoyed sparingly. Coffee is fine with heavy cream or black, as is tea. But, of course, you should avoid adding sugar. See the "Bulletproof Coffee" recipe at the end of the book.

You can even indulge in an alcoholic beverage. Many "hard" liquors don't have carbs. But stay away from the fruity drinks (margaritas, daiquiris, rum punch, and any others that taste sweet) and tonic, which contains a lot of sugar. Instead, order a vodka with seltzer and a twist of lime or something similar.

Build a Good System of Support and Accountability

I wrote this book to make it as close as possible to the experience you would have if you were to come to my weight management center. But one necessary thing that can't be replicated in a book is accountability. In my program, the weigh-ins are important because they help keep my patients on track. No one wants to come in without having lost any weight. And they definitely don't want to see any weight gain. That kind of positive peer pressure helps, too. So I recommend you ask a friend or a family member you trust to weigh you in each week. Every Sunday screenshot a picture of your weight from the app you are using or just take a picture of the scale while you are weighing yourself and send it to your friend or family member. Maybe you can do that for one another. Being accountable to someone other than yourself will help keep you on the straight and narrow. The NGW app does that, as well.

Building a good system of support and accountability is important at this stage. Most people are super motivated when they first decide to make a lifestyle change and lose weight, but maintaining that motivation is another story. A bad day or even a bad moment can change everything. It helps to have someone to lean on in those times. Studies have shown that people are more successful losing weight if they find a partner or more to join them. I recommend that you let people know what you are doing to try to change your life so that your support network can help keep you motivated. In my clinic we provide that motivation (almost like a cheerleader) to help patients keep going. My patients participate in a support group, where we meet to discuss challenges, celebrate successes, share ideas, inspire those who need it, and more. If someone is struggling in a particular area, there's usually someone else in the group who has been there and can share a strategy for success, or at the very least, offer some encouragement.

I understand that many people just can't make it to those meetings, including many readers, so I've also created an online community to fill the gap. You may join the support group so you, too, can communicate with others who are on this journey. To join the online community, check out Facebook for the group (No Guesswork). Participating in a virtual support group can be almost as effective as attending meetings in person, but the key is engagement. To find the support you are seeking, you must chime in and let the members know who you are. Of course, exercise the same caution you would when you participate in any online community by not divulging anything confidential. But it is a group of people who are trying to navigate their way together to healthier lives. I participate in the group as often as possible, and so it's the next best thing to visiting my clinic. There's no cost to join. We do our best to hold your hand through this journey.

If you're the type of person who will be more accountable to someone you know and trust, ask a friend to join you on the entire journey. Then, the two of you can set up the terms for how to keep one another accountable. Will you meet in person or check in by email or text? Will you weigh yourself weekly and reveal your weight changes (not necessarily your weight) to one another? Whatever you decide, just know that you don't have to do it alone.

Increase Sleep, Decrease Stress

Sleep is important, more than just for mental health reasons. Remember ghrelin, (the Hunger Gremlin)? If you don't get the appropriate sleep, the Hunger Gremlin grows (meaning your ghrelin level increases). You are then much more likely to feel famished and to get off track with your eating. People with untreated sleep apnea are very susceptible to increased ghrelin levels, which leaves them hungry and craving carbs throughout the day. Studies show that shift workers, particularly those working the overnight shift, also have higher rates of obesity. Lack of sleep is a likely culprit. So, make sure you get a good amount of sleep, which for most people is seven to eight hours on average.

Stress also increases ghrelin (as well as cortisol) and ultimately, insulin, thereby increasing fat storage. So, I recommend you participate in activities that reduce your stress, such as yoga, exercise, reading a good book, watching a movie, spending time with family and friends, or any other safe activity that helps you to relax. But if you continue to feel stressed on a regular basis, you may need to seek professional counseling. Often, when I ask people why they think they are struggling with obesity, they say things, like "I eat too much," or "I eat a lot of junk," or "I eat too much of the wrong things." But I tell them, that's not really the problem; that's how they choose to treat the problem. So, the goal is to find out what the real problem is. What is causing you stress? What is causing you to feel anxious? Are you using food to treat your anxiety? Are you emotional eating because you are having problems at home or on the job, and food is a familiar comfort? Are you feeling depressed? Many times, overeating is just a symptom of a broader problem. What needs to be fixed is the thing that is causing you to turn to food. Addressing the underlying issue is beyond the scope of this book, but I want you to think about what those issues may be and, if needed, seek professional help to address them. Doing so is critical to your long-term success.

As a doctor, I always think about primary prevention (stopping something before it starts), as well. So, I advise you to try your best to avoid stressful situations. Whether at work or home, strategize to make your environment as pleasant (stress-free) as possible. You don't have to be ready for war at work all the time or win every argument at home. Pursue peace.

Snack Sensibly

It's okay if you like to snack between meals. Actually, I even encourage it; it keeps the Hunger Gremlin away. You just have to be sensible about it, and that means you should choose proteins and fats. There are lots of great options. Here are some popular protein snacks:

- ★ Protein Shake (Make sure it has less than 10 grams of carbs.)
- ★ Beef jerky
- ★ Boiled eggs
- ★ Egg Muffins
- ★ Cheese sticks
- ★ Snack-size peanut butter
- ★ Celery sticks (Try it with peanut butter or plain)
- ★ Rolled turkey slices
- ★ Pecans/Brazil nuts/macadamia nuts/peanuts/walnuts/almonds/ (Be sure to check the carb content per serving.)
- ★ Plain Greek yogurt with a tablespoon of blueberries (Be careful to check the carb content; some brands are loaded with sugar.)
- ★ Cottage cheese
- ★ Protein chips (If you like potato chips, these tasty crisps come in a variety of flavors, such as barbeque and sour cream and onion.)
- ★ Portable protein packs (Some food companies are creating on-the-go packs with nuts, cheese pieces, and deli meat cubes)
- ★ Chaffles (a low-carb option for waffles and bread)

Here are some great high-fat, low-carb snacks:

★ Guacamole
★ Cheese dip
★ Pork rinds
★ Deviled eggs
★ Parmesan cheese crisps/wisps
★ Spinach dip (Try spinach dip with Tortilla-style protein chips, instead of Tortilla chips.)
★ Turkey pepperoni
★ Protein Snack packs

Here are some other low-carb snacks:

★ Dill Pickles
★ Cucumber slices
★ Olives
★ Mini-carrots with ranch dressing
★ Kale chips

Maintain a Winning Attitude

Attitude is so important when you're trying to lose weight and, more importantly, change your life. You first have to believe that you can do it, that you can thrive on a low-carb diet in this high-carb world. Carbs are not going away anytime soon. But with a winning attitude, you are confident in your ability to manage them and stay on track. You know that you are worth the sacrifices you are making to reach your goal. And sacrifice is not a dirty word. In fact, getting healthier is not much of a sacrifice at all.

If your goal is to lose weight, picture in your mind how you want to look. Pull out a favorite old photograph of yourself at the size you want to be and post it in a prominent place or as the home screen on your cell phone as a constant reminder of what you are trying to achieve. With a winning attitude, you will use that vision of where you want to be to push yourself forward, not to condemn yourself for being overweight.

A winning attitude is fueled by hope and positivity. So pay attention to the thoughts that creep into your mind and the words that come out of your mouth. Try to eliminate any negative thoughts with positive affirmations that remind yourself that you are on a life-changing journey and that getting where you want to be will take time. You didn't get where you are overnight, and so you can't turn it around overnight. Remind yourself that you are on the right track and headed in the right direction. Often, it's easier to show kindness and give encouragement to someone else than it is to be kind to ourselves. But we need to do it. What would you say to encourage your best friend? Well, try saying the same things to yourself.

I have patients who stop losing weight or a few who may have even gained some weight. And it really bums them out. They are baffled why I'm not worried about it. Well, I'm worried about it, but not really that much. And do you know why? Because as long as they keep coming, as long as they keep showing up, as long as they keep caring, they will start losing weight again. I will make sure of it. The same is true for you. If you show up, you will get to a healthier weight, and you will reach your goal. This reminds me of my dad, who battled drug addiction for much of his life. Every time that he relapsed he said to me confidently, "Don't worry. I will get it together." And I knew he would because he was so determined, no matter how many times he failed. And you know what? He finally did conquer his addiction.

This weight loss battle is won or lost first in your mind. Does having a winning attitude mean that you never feel down or that you never fail? Not at all. It just means that you don't quit, that you find a way to rise up when you slip down. It means that if you veer off course, you quickly find your way back on track. You don't dwell on your mistakes. You don't beat yourself up. You get up and hit that reset button. You learn whatever lesson is to be learned and keep moving forward. Each step forward moves you closer to your destination.

NEAT Way To Increase Physical Activity

By now, you know all about the eating part, and you're wondering about exercise. Should you do it? And if so, how much? The short answers are yes, you absolutely should increase your physical activity, and you should do so as often as possible. Notice that I said "physical activity," and not just "exercise." I'll explain that shortly. In my clinic, we try to get the diet right first before we start discussing physical activity because, as I've said, what you eat is *the* most important factor in losing weight and keeping it off. Unfortunately, we are taught that exercise is the key to weight loss, and that is a very flawed concept. Think about it: if you exercise for a solid hour, you burn maybe 200 to 300 calories per session. If you're killing it in the gym, you might burn 500 calories. But that is of little value if you are not watching what you eat. Remember the 80-20 rule? Eighty percent of weight loss is based on what you put in your mouth, and 20 percent is based on physical activity.

That said, let's take full advantage of the 20 percent. Moving your body burns calories, and the more you burn, the fewer calories are left to be stored as fat. Plus, exercise has a host of other health benefits. It puts you in a better mood by releasing endorphins, chemicals that produce positive feelings and decrease depression. Studies of people with diagnosed depression have shown that exercise at any level significantly decreases feelings of depression. So that alone is a great benefit. But exercise also helps to build muscles, strengthen bones, decrease insulin resistance, and promote a healthy heart. Let's get moving.

There are certain rules that you have to follow before embarking on an exercise regime. Rule number one: Don't hurt yourself! Rule number two: Don't hurt yourself! Rule number three: Don't hurt yourself! I find that my patients are often so excited about finally losing weight that they want to get in the gym right away. We think that's what we are supposed to do. That's what we see the healthy people in the TV ads doing. But if you've been totally inactive, it is much better to start slowly. That's why I want you to shed 10-, 20-, 30- pounds first, depending, of course, on how much you have to lose. Your safety is my primary concern. Say if someone all of a sudden threw a 30-pound vest on your back and told you to go running and do a High Intensity Interval Training (HIIT) exercise program. You would hurt yourself for sure. You have to be at a high level of fitness to perform that kind of workout safely. So, we start with the first step, getting the weight off. I want you to increase your physical activity, but that does not necessarily mean that you should rush to the gym. There are so many other ways you can become more physically active and derive the same, if not greater, health benefits.

In science, we call the energy you burn when you're not sleeping, eating, working out in a gym, or doing any planned exercise Non-Exercise Activity Thermogenesis (NEAT). Think about it. There are 168 hours in a week. The average person who exercises might do so up to five times a week, so let's say five hours a week (and someone going to the gym five times a week is killing it, as they say). Either way, that leaves another 163 hours, and if you subtract the forty-nine hours that we are supposed to spend sleeping, that still leaves 114 hours of wakefulness that we can use to expend more energy and burn more calories—114 hours of NEAT, compared to five hours of exercise. So, if you maximize your NEAT, it adds up. Research shows that you can burn 30 percent more calories with NEAT than with exercise alone, and that makes sense, given the tremendous number of hours we spend doing things other than working out.

So, how do you increase your NEAT? It's really pretty simple. Think extra. Add something extra to the things you do every single day. For example, instead of circling the parking lot in your vehicle to look for the closest space to your favorite store in the mall, find a space at the far end of the parking lot or garage and walk further. It's usually pretty empty down there anyway. A few of my patients have asked me for a disability parking placard so they can park their vehicles close to the door everywhere they go. But I don't allow them to use obesity as an excuse not to move more, and I say a resounding no! Unless you really need it, of course. Because I want them to park further away and walk. I want you to take the stairs instead of the elevator. If you work on the sixth floor and can't walk up six flights of stairs, walk up as many as you can and take the elevator for the rest. Or start by walking down the stairs first. Walk to lunch during your break instead of driving around the corner to Subway. One of my patients actually moved her printer from a side corner of her desk to a space across the room so that she would have to get up and walk every time she used the printer. And she used the printer a lot, which meant she was up and out of her chair a lot!

If there's a water cooler next to your desk and one on the other side of the building, I want you to walk to the one on the other side of the building. I want you to move more! Get your NEAT up!

In the airport, skip the People Mover and walk from gate to gate. At home, get on the floor and play with the kids or grandkids, or take them out to the yard to throw a ball or play tag instead of sitting in a chair to watch them play. Walk up the stairs to talk to your son or daughter instead of standing at the foot of the stairs and yelling your message. Give the gardener a break and pull your own weeds or mow your own grass. Sweep, mop, and dust more often. Tap your feet and lift your legs while you are sitting on the sofa watching TV. Put on some good music and move your body while you're washing dishes. It may sound ridiculous, but it's not. The point is you can burn many more calories by finding ways to get extra mileage out of your routine activities. If you think of every bit of effort as a penny, every penny counts and pennies add up. Get your NEAT up!

For those of you who have been to the gym in the past year and feel comfortable that you can work out safely, feel free to add a gym workout to your routine at least three to four times a week. But before you embark on any workout plan, make sure you check with your doctor first. Take advantage of the gym's personnel to help you figure out a routine that combines aerobic activity—treadmill, elliptical, bicycle, etc.—and some type of weight or resistance training that helps to build muscle. Sign up for a fitness class that you like—line dancing, hip hop, cycling, step aerobics, jazzercise, Zumba, yoga, the list goes on. People tend to be more consistent if they find an activity they enjoy. Workouts in the water are popular, too, especially if you have bad knees or suffer from other joint pain. Most gyms offer exercise classes in the pool, but you can also go to the local YMCA and do your own simple routines, like walking from one side of the pool to the other several times, adding some squats, and kicking as you hold onto the side of the pool. If you're a swimmer, swim a few laps. It's a great aerobic activity, and it's gentle on your joints. If you prefer working out at home, go to YouTube, which has an abundance of any kind of workout you can imagine. If you have the desire, the options to increase your physical activity—on any budget or no budget at all—are limitless.

Desire is key. If technology is an indicator, we don't really desire to move much. Despite all of its great benefits, technology has made us lazier. Our gadgets do many of the things we used to expend energy to do. We don't have to walk through the house to turn out our lights any more, we set electronic timers, use an app, or voice commands. We don't even have to walk to the computer to type a question into Google for an answer to a burning question; we can ask Alexa (or whatever your device's name is) from the comfort of our recliner. The indoor mall is quickly becoming a thing of the past. There's very little browsing from one end of the mall to the next these days. We want to park right outside our favorite store, dash in and out and drive to the next one. And many of us don't even bother going to the store. Amazon delivers our clothes and our groceries. Or if we prefer, we just have to pull our vehicle into the delivery lanes at Walmart while we're out, and the groceries we ordered while we were sitting at our computer or on our phone are loaded into the trunks of our vehicles. Or we can ask Alexa for groceries: we just sit on our couch and say, "Alexa order me some paper towels." We are now living out what at one time was considered a futuristic movie. One day in the not too distant future, we won't even have to use up energy to give a voice command; we'll just use our thoughts to make our desires a reality, like in the 2008 Pixar movie, *WALL-E*. Don't get me wrong: I'm not knocking convenience. We live in a fast-paced world, and we're all busier than we've ever been. But the down side is this: we're sitting more. And sitting has become the new smoking. It's helping to make us have more obesity and to be sicker.

So, don't let the convenience of technology stop you from moving. Find ways to push yourself to move more, and if necessary, shut down some of that technology every now and then to force yourself to get out of your seat. Moving more will make you feel more inspired to stay on track. It helps to create a healthy mindset. You will have a greater desire to eat right because you will not want to feel that the time spent working out or increasing your physical activity was wasted. But here's the key: don't compare yourself to anyone else. You are your only competition. Do your personal best and keep pushing yourself to do more. It is a permanent lifestyle change that you are trying to create. Remember this isn't a sprint; it's a well-paced journey to becoming your best self. And most important of all, you are positioning yourself to win.

CHAPTER EIGHT

PHASE TWO

Preparing For Landing

Congratulations! You've lost 10 percent of your body weight, which means you have finished Phase One of the NGW plan! This is a huge milestone, and you should feel very proud of yourself. Losing 10 percent of your body weight is what we medical professionals call "clinically meaningful weight loss." When patients achieve clinically meaningful weight loss, they start to see changes in their overall health (blood pressure improves, blood sugar is better regulated, joint pains lessen, and more). So, you should start experiencing some of these improvements. If you are taking any medications, you need to see your doctor (if you haven't already), so that he or she can determine whether you should stop taking the medications or reduce them.

Many doctors would tell you at this stage that you've achieved what is considered a reasonable expectation for weight loss. Expecting to lose much more is considered an unreasonable expectation for most people to do on their own. But losing more weight is not unreasonable if you stick to the NGW plan. That's the purpose of this book—to help you develop a lifestyle that will change your life forever. And yes, that includes reaching your weight loss goal, regardless of what it is. You can get there if you stay focused and stick to the plan.

Even if you decide you are satisfied with your 10 percent weight loss, your next goal should be to maintain it. You don't want the effort you put into losing the weight to be in vain. You are now a healthier person, and I want to help you keep it that way. The details of the maintenance phase are outlined a bit later in the book, and you can skip ahead if you'd like. If you want to lose more weight, though, let's keep moving forward toward your goal.

Phase Two is similar to Phase One, with just a few tweaks. You have mastered staying below your carb number; you know how to do this. You're almost an expert. So, let's just work on a little fine-tuning.

Make Sure Your Low-Carb Diet Is Well-Balanced

At this stage, you've cut many carbs out of your diet and you should be feeling really good, physically and mentally. You should be moving better, sleeping better, and in an overall better mood. So, now it's time to make sure your low-carb diet is well-formulated.

What are you eating? I know you are eating low-carb foods because you are staying under your personalized carb number and losing weight. But are you eating a well-formulated low-carb diet? And what does that mean, exactly? This may surprise you, but the best formulated low-carb diet should be full of healthy fat (yes, don't be scared!). As a matter of fact, healthy fats should make up the majority of your diet (60-80 percent). You should consume moderate amounts of protein (20-30 percent) and a low amount of carbohydrates (5-10 percent).

A Well-Formulated Low-Carb Diet

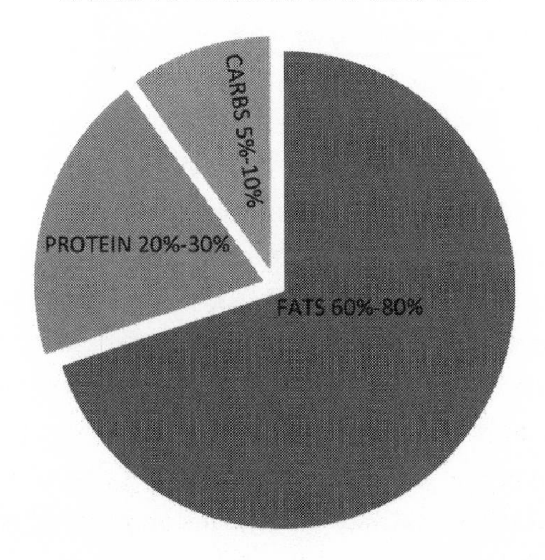

I didn't mention this in the beginning because I wanted to give you time to get accustomed to a low-carb lifestyle before I threw something else at you. One thing at a time.

The other reason I didn't explain the well-formulated low-carb diet earlier is I truly didn't want to scare you. Fat has an undeserved bad reputation. As I explained in the beginning of this book, we've been taught our entire lives that fat makes us fat and that we should shun it, even though the science is clear that it just isn't true. I laid out the science for you earlier in this book. Yet still, when you hear that fat should make up the biggest part of your healthy, low-carb diet, it's tough for you to believe. But I'm asking you to trust the process.

Don't Believe The Hype (It's crazy)

People will tell you that the things you've read in this book aren't true, and they won't have any evidence. But you do! You can provide them with the evidence that I have provided you in this book. They will argue that losing weight is all about willpower. Just direct them to the latest studies on the physiology of gut hormones and how they affect and control hunger and cravings. Or, better yet, just tell them to read this book. It amazes me that as a society we have been doing this diet thing the same way (pushing a low-fat diet for weight loss) for fifty years, yet obesity continues to get worse year after year. That sounds like the definition of insanity to me, doing the same thing over and over, yet expecting different results.

There is also what psychologists called cognitive dissonance, the mental discomfort (psychological stress) experienced by a person who simultaneously holds two or more contradictory beliefs, ideas, or values. This discomfort is triggered when a person's belief clashes with new evidence to the contrary. When confronted with the contradictory facts that challenge their personal beliefs, ideals, and values, people often try to find ways to resolve the matter and reduce their discomfort. Sound familiar?

The "experts" have tried for decades to explain why the low-fat craze didn't produce the expected results. They say people just don't have enough willpower. They say it's all a matter of exercise. But their beliefs and explanations just aren't congruent with the facts. It's cognitive dissonance. Or as

I like to say, willful ignorance of the facts. But you know better. Now, you can do better.

Avoid Eating Late

Before now, I've said nothing about *when* to eat. But remember, we're fine-tuning now. When you eat can have a major effect on your weight loss; case in point: late-night eating.

Consider this patient of mine who came back for a follow-up weight management visit. She was super frustrated. She'd been doing everything right, she said, following the plan as she always had. Yet, her weight loss had stalled suddenly. When weight loss stops, there is ALWAYS a reason. Usually, the culprits are hidden carbs or too much protein (yes, you can actually eat too much protein!). But sometimes, neither is the case. My patient was adamant that she was keeping her carbs at or below her goal of 60 grams per day on average for the week. Because she was tracking faithfully, I was able to look through her diary in her app and, sure enough, her carb count was in the 40s or 50s pretty much every day. So I pressed her a bit on the hidden carbs. She said that because I had told her about them before, she was always looking out for hidden carbs. She accounted for any sauce she put on her meat, and if she couldn't figure out how many carbs were in the sauce, she wouldn't eat it. She wouldn't eat anything with carbs that couldn't be counted. Plus, she stayed well under her personalized number of 60 to build in a little cushion for the hidden carbs. That's what frustrated her the most. She was working so hard but still not losing weight. She wasn't gaining weight either, but she just couldn't understand why the things that worked for her in the beginning didn't seem to be working now.

I moved to the next questions in my assessment. Was it possible that she was eating too much protein? Did she have a well-formulated low-carb diet? I examined her diary again, and yep, her fat intake percentage was at 60 percent most days. I was also measuring her muscle composition, and I noticed that she had lost a couple of pounds of muscle on her last body composition test, and so I didn't think she was eating too much protein. As a matter of fact, I told her she needed to eat a bit more protein, since she seemed to be losing muscle. But that didn't explain the sudden stall in her weight loss. What was it? It had to be something. And then something popped in her head. She was a teacher. It was summertime, and her schedule was different than it had been during the school year. During the school year, she ate dinner around 6 p.m. so that she could get to bed earlier and be well-rested for school the next day. With a more relaxed schedule, dinner was now later, around 8 p.m. or 9 p.m. That was likely it! We'd cracked the code, I told her. I asked her to OSCC- make one simple consistent change: go back to eating earlier in the evening. She did just that, and when she returned three weeks later, she was down five pounds. She was astonished! Nothing else changed, just the time she ate dinner. And she made sure she didn't eat anything else after that. She asked the question many of you may want to know: Why does the time we eat make such a big difference in weight loss? Because of what I call the Bonnie and Clyde of hormones.

Bonnie (Insulin) is the fat storage hormone, and you have to keep her levels low, or she and her conniving partner, Clyde (ghrelin, aka The Hunger Gremlin), will cause havoc. Studies have shown that if you eat the same meal at noon versus 10 p.m., Bonnie will spike significantly higher at 10 p.m., thereby increasing your fat storage. Under those conditions, your body can't burn fat because when Bonnie is high, she holds energy hostage, essentially keeping it locked in the fat cells. The result is fat storage and likely weight gain. Or, in my patient's case, the fat-burning, weight loss cycle came to a sudden halt.

When people stop losing weight on my plan, there's always a reason. If my patients stop losing weight and declare they're doing everything that they are supposed to do, I go through a battery of tests, as I did with the patient above to find out what is going on. Most times, I don't do these tests for me; I do these tests for them. And unlike with my patient above, most times, people stop losing weight because they stopped being as strict and disciplined as they were in the beginning. But they've fooled themselves into thinking that if they are doing close to what they were doing when they started, they should be okay. Close is only good, however, if you're playing horseshoes. This is when I have them do the Hunt Motivational Scale (HMS that we discussed in Chapter 5) with me in the office. So if your weight lose stalls I advise you to go back and do the HMS as well. It will help you hone in on where your issues are. That way you can focus on that area to get your score back up and the weight loss will resume. Here's the tough truth: This program is an all-or-none phenomenon. If you do it, it works; if you don't do it, it doesn't work. Period. Even if you "kinda" do it (meaning you eat just a little bit over your personalized number), it won't work. You have to follow the program for it to work. To continue losing weight, you have to continue being the committed person you were in the beginning. Make sure you are still tracking everything and planning your meals.

Consider Intermittent Fasting

Another eating pattern has the same physiology as low-carb eating; it's known as intermittent fasting. With intermittent fasting, you alternate periods of eating and fasting. There are various methods of intermittent fasting, including one popular method in which you fast for sixteen hours, restricting eating to a period of eight hours. It's not as tough as it may sound. In that scenario, you could eat between, say, noon and 8 p.m. (or 11 a.m. and 7 p.m. or 10 a.m. and 6 p.m.), essentially skipping breakfast (or eating a late breakfast), following your regular low-carb meal plan during those eight hours, and eating nothing after that designated eighth hour. You are asleep for the vast majority of the time that you are fasting. Many people I know who have tried intermittent fasting prefer that method for that very reason—you are sleeping for the vast majority of the fasting time. And remember, you also don't want to get an insulin spike late at night from eating after hours.

Other common methods include whole-day fasts (24 hours of fasting, followed by 24 hours of eating regularly), or five days of non-fasting followed by two days of fasting. The effects on the body are essentially the same; you just have to choose a method that is most comfortable for you.

Intermittent fasting is good because it works the same as a well-formulated low-carb diet; they both keep your insulin level low. The goal is to lower your insulin, to not just lose weight but keep it off by reducing or eliminating insulin resistance, which is the main cause of the weight-gaining cycle. An insulin spike is one thing, but a constant high level of insulin produces more visceral fat (fatty liver and other fat in your belly), which then produces more insulin resistance, further increasing insulin, which further increases fat cells, and the cycle continues year after year. That cycle causes a weight gain of one to two pounds on average every year. As I mentioned earlier in this book, as a nation, we are not eating more calories or exercising less. So why are we developing more and more obesity? Insulin resistance. The more insulin resistant we become, the more obesity we develop, and the more insulin we continue to produce. Diabetes (type 2) is primarily caused by insulin resistance and obesity; in some medical circles, the disease is known as "diabesity." In my clinic, we proudly say that we *cure*, not just treat, diabetes. And we do that with a high-fat, low-carb diet that decreases insulin production. You can get a similar effect with intermittent fasting.

Critics of intermittent fasting say it's not sustainable, but I've heard the same criticism about low-carb diets. It may seem unsustainable because it requires discipline. But now that you have made it to Phase Two, you've shown that you are serious and disciplined. So, if you want to give it a try, intermittent fasting may enhance your success. Just make sure that when you eat during non-fasting hours, you continue eating a low-carb diet. You can't get around keeping your carbs low because in doing so, you keep your insulin low. If you try intermittent fasting simply because you want to eat carbs during the time you are not fasting, it's not going to work. Your insulin level will spike, and those spikes will make it difficult for you to lose the weight, not to mention it will keep you hungry. That, of course, is not good for periods of fasting. I believe one of the main reasons some say intermittent fasting isn't sustainable is because many people fill up on carbs during the non-fasting hours. Remember, a high-carb diet not only causes a spike in your insulin, but it causes you to crave more carbs, and the cycle repeats.

Whether or not you try intermittent fasting is a personal choice. It is not a requirement of Phase Two, but rather another tool that may help you reach your weight loss goal and maintain it. If you are satisfied with the progress of your weight loss so far, you may want to stay on track by just keeping your carbs below your personalized number. But if your weight loss has slowed a bit, intermittent fasting may add an extra spark. The main side effect of intermittent fasting is the same as what you may experience on a low-carb diet: the "keto flu" (or as I call it, "keto dehydration"). But by now, you know what to do, just drink some bone broth (best) or bouillon soup.

If you choose not to do intermittent fasting, you still must pay close attention to meal timing to keep your insulin level low. You should allow at least twelve hours from your last meal until you eat breakfast (or break fast). So, if you eat your last meal at 6 p.m., you can eat breakfast as early as 6 a.m., and you have given your body time for the insulin to drop to its lowest level and fat-burning to churn at its highest level. Depending on your schedule, you can eat at 7 p.m. or even 8 p.m., as long as roughly twelve hours elapse before you eat again (7 a.m. or 8 a.m.). Eating much later than 8 p.m. has negative effects on insulin and can cause fat production. During those twelve hours of fasting, you should eat nothing and drink only water.

Try a Carb Detox (If Needed)

What if you have a bad week or weeks? Don't beat yourself up. You've made it to Phase Two, and so you know the plan works. The train is moving in the right direction; you just have to get back on it. And the quicker you do so, the less time it will take you to recover lost time.

A three-day carb detox may help you hit the reset button. The process is very simple: To do a three-day carb detox, you just have to get your carbs extremely low, less than 50 grams per day (actually in the 20's, 30's, or 40's each day). Do this for three days, and it will reset your brain, drop your insulin level, and help you readjust. Afterwards, beginning on Day 4, you can go back to your personalized carb number and expect the weight loss to begin again.

Don't Take the Rest Stop

When I was in medical school, two of my best friends and I took a trip to Las Vegas. Once there, we decided to rent a car and travel to Los Angeles. It was an interesting trip. I will spare you the details except to say that when we got on Interstate 10, it felt like the longest drive of my life. The highway was straight with no curves or turns; there were no stores, no gas stations, nothing but desert and tumbleweeds on both sides. I wouldn't have survived if it wasn't for my friends, who kept the journey entertaining.

I liken your journey of getting to a healthier weight to my I-10 road trip from Las Vegas to L.A., except there may be no friends in the car with you. It's just you, and your radio isn't even working. This is Phase Two, the longest part of your journey. Sometimes it seems monotonous, maybe even boring.

Imagine you get closer to your destination, close enough to see city lights in the distance, and out of nowhere you see flashing lights that read "rest stop." You've been on this long journey of weight loss, just you and your thoughts. You're tired. You may even be a little bored. Those flashing lights—a place to stop and put the journey on hold—look pretty enticing. Why not stop? Because of this: people who exit at the rest stop tend to never leave. They stall, and never get to their destination; their goal weight. Or if they do leave the rest stop and get back on the highway, they go a little further down the road and turn right back around to return to that rest stop, entering a state of what I call quasi-maintenance. I've seen this too often in my clinic. Quasi-maintenance is when they're not gaining any weight, but they're also not actively losing any weight, either, and they've become somewhat comfortable with that.

If you're in quasi-maintenance and you'd like to shift into Maintenance Phase for now, that's fine. The Maintenance Phase is a different strategy than active weight loss; we will discuss that in a later chapter. But make a decision to actively go down one path or the other. Why? Because quasi-maintenance is a "no-man's land" of eating, where you're setting yourself up for failure. People in quasi-maintenance tend to start regaining after a short period of time. Before long, they have gained ten to twenty pounds.

I learned that quasi-maintenance is no good the hard way, from working with patients. I've seen that motivating patients to leave the rest stop once they've stopped there is one of the hardest things to do. Their momentum is lost and they can't seem to get it back. Why? It may be due to discouragement. Too many times, when patients stop just short of their goal, they stay a little too long and get discouraged, and then start traveling back in the opposite direction. Then, it's just a matter of time before their weight starts to rise. And they end up right back at their set point, their starting weight. In that case, your body won. Your body is happy. And you don't have to worry about anything because your body is no longer trying to fight you, so you don't have to think about this anymore. But you are back to an unhealthy weight, and all the things that go along with it.

Now, for the sake of comparison, consider the experience of another person taking this same journey—same deal, desert on either side with tumbleweeds everywhere, and a busted radio. But this person's mindset is different. He's not feeling bored, alone, or tired, rolling along the highway. He's über excited, counting the mile markers (i.e., pounds lost) whizzing past, anticipating the thrill of reaching his destination (his goal weight). He, too, notices the rest stop seemingly pop out of nowhere, but he blows right past it without a second thought. Why? Well, why would he stop? He has only ten more miles to go to get to his destination. He's made so much progress to get this far; he knows the rest stop is only a delay and a distraction.

Those are the different mindsets I encounter all the time. Which person are you? I want you to be the person who keeps going, the one who realizes there's no real rest in a "rest stop." It's nothing but a hindrance. My advice to you is the same: Don't stop! Don't be fooled by the flashing lights, beckoning you to take a break. And if, by chance, you've already made that stop, leave immediately! All is not lost. Keep going towards your goal. You're almost there!

Wear It Like A Crown

One of the amazing things about this lifestyle change is the "halo effect." When people see you losing weight, they're going to want to know how you did it. Then you're going to start noticing people around you doing what you're doing and losing weight, as well. That is a huge compliment to you, to your commitment and discipline. So, wear your success like a crown. You've earned this glory! Know that you're not the only one to benefit from your lifestyle change. Now, you're serving as a shining example for friends, family, and any others who want to know a healthy way to achieve their weight goals.

CHAPTER NINE

Losing To Win

When I first met William "Bill" Reeves Jr., he was 39 years old, 456 pounds, and concerned about a large red bruise on his lower leg. He assumed the bruise was related to his weight, and he just wanted to get it checked out—at least, that's what he told me. I would learn later that the bruise was perhaps an excuse; the real reason he'd come to see me was much deeper.

As age 40 crept closer, Bill had become more reflective about his life. He realized he was feeling anxious and depressed, thinking about all of the things he could no longer do because of his weight. Standing nearly six feet, two inches tall, Bill had always been a "big boy." Even as a sophomore in high school, he had weighed about 250 pounds. But in high school and college, being big had its advantages. Bill played football, he was active and muscular, and he used his weight to crush guys on the playing field. But in the years after college, he gradually gained more and more weight and became less and less active. With his 40th birthday looming, he started thinking of what he could do to guard against the impending doom. He wondered: What if he could lose weight? He mentioned the idea to his father, who happened to be a patient of mine in my general practice at the time. His father loved that Bill was thinking seriously about trying to lose weight and told him about my then-new weight management clinic.

On Bill's first visit, I examined the bruise, which turned out to be minor, despite its appearance. The bruise also had nothing to do with his weight, but Bill knew it was finally time for him to face the real reason he'd come in seeking help. He had struggled with many other attempts to shed the pounds, but he was in a different place emotionally this time. His desire to lose weight was more serious. He was ready to change.

Bill's Journey Begins

During that first visit, I shared with Bill a fact about his weight that he had never heard before: it was not his fault. I explained that I wasn't just trying to make him feel better but that there were real scientific reasons why it had been difficult for him to shed the pounds, and more importantly, why it was so difficult to keep them off. I described how carbs light up the craving center and make you want to eat more carbs. I also explained how the human body resists and works against us when we lose weight, how our system literally shuts down our metabolism to get back to a weight it perceives as normal (the set point). As a social policy researcher, Bill is a smart guy, a natural thinker and problem solver, and so the science just made sense to him.

"I have a few tools in my toolbox," I told him. "If this one doesn't work, we'll move to the next one." Those simple words were reassuring to Bill. He told me later that knowing he had options made him feel less threatened by the mountainous task before him. My approach was purposeful. Even though I knew Bill would face serious, life-threatening health consequences in the future if he didn't lose weight, I didn't want to put that kind of pressure on him. So I avoided the "do this or die" scenario. I wanted him to know this was a journey that we would take together, that I would guide him every step of the way, and that we would make adjustments, as needed.

I started with a baseline question: What was he eating? There was just one way to know for sure. He had to begin tracking everything he ate. The other instructions were also pretty simple: he could eat until he felt full, but he should keep his carbs below 100 grams per day (with a target of 75 grams). To keep his expectations realistic, I set a weight loss goal of one to two pounds a week, which is the average amount of weight a participant can expect to lose under my plan. Bill's next appointment would be in two weeks—a schedule we would maintain throughout his journey.

When Bill showed up for his follow-up visit two weeks later, he stepped on the scale and got a big surprise. He had exceeded his weight loss goal by shedding five pounds. We both were ecstatic! This was just a pebble from the mountain he had to move, but now he knew something he hadn't been sure of before: that the mountain *could* move. He just had to keep chipping away at it. The psychological impact of that small accomplishment was huge for Bill. He said it felt as if a switch flipped on in his brain, and from that moment on, he just kept knocking off the pebbles—one, or two, or a few at a time. At every checkup, his weight went down, and it just kept decreasing.

In the first year, Bill lost 185 pounds. Then he lost another 40-plus pounds over several months, dropping to a new low weight of 225 pounds, about equal to the amount of weight that he'd lost. Bill lost half his size without medicine or surgery! Now, let me pause here and say that as proud as I am of Bill, I realize that everyone has a different journey and needs different tools to help them reach his/her destination. About 50 to 60 percent of my patients need an additional tool from my toolbox, medication. If they want to start with just the NGW dietary plan, we do that, but if I see that a patient is really struggling to stay on task (most of my patients have been trying to lose weight all their lives before they show up at my doorstep), I revisit the idea of an anti-obesity medication (approved by the Food and Drug Administration (FDA) for safety and effectiveness) to suppress hunger and cravings. Some of my patients, like Bill, insist that they do not want to take any medicines, but I do my best to assure that there is no guilt associated with needing additional help. It's just another tool in my toolbox. According to FDA rules, a patient with a Body Mass Index (BMI) greater than 30 or a BMI of 27 with an associated health condition can qualify for a prescription. Remember your body is working against you to get you back to the weight that it perceives as normal by increasing ghrelin and decreasing the satiating hormones that make you feel satisfied and keep you from overeating. These FDA-approved medicines counteract that by either fighting the ghrelin or providing an actual satiating hormone. So medication is an option that you, too, can discuss with your doctor if you are unable to succeed on the meal plan alone because of overwhelming hunger and cravings.

Think of taking medication for weight loss as similar to taking something for high blood pressure. If your blood pressure was high, you'd be willing to take a medication to get it to a lower healthier number. Why? Because you know that getting your blood pressure down reduces your risk of stroke and heart attack. You also know that getting to a healthier weight reduces your risk of diabetes and hypertension (which can lead to strokes and heart attacks), and that it decreases your risk of different cancers, blood clots, and many other things, as well. In fact, an argument can be made that getting your weight down reduces your risk of developing an array of medical conditions to a greater degree than reducing your blood pressure alone. So we approach treating obesity along the same lines as treating high blood pressure in that *if you need* medications, we will prescribe them to reduce your health risk, as we would with high blood pressure.

The Medical Tools for Weight Loss

The development of multiple safe, effective medications is among some of the newer advancements in obesity medicine. Since 2012, the FDA has approved four new weight loss drugs and there are more being considered for approval at this present time. Three of them are pills, and another is available in injectable form. The drugs work with a kind of one-two punch by blocking the effects of the gut hormone (ghrelin) that triggers hunger and cravings, while simultaneously stimulating the receptors that signal satiety. Interestingly, three of the drugs have already been FDA-approved for other uses. Two are oral combination therapies and one is an injectable that was previously approved to treat type 2 diabetes. One such combination mixes a common anti-depressant that has been shown to cause weight loss by working on the craving and hunger centers in your brain for a brief period with another drug that is used to counteract the effects of an opioid overdose. The mixture enables the anti-depressant to work more effectively to aid in weight loss. The other oral medication mixes a medication used to treat migraine headaches and epilepsy with an amphetamine-derived appetite suppressant. Someone taking these medications feels full for longer periods, not experiencing the powerful urges to eat. Another positive is that the drugs have minimal side effects and are generally well-tolerated by most people. But let me stress this point: any such medications should be prescribed and monitored only by your physician. Please do not attempt to diagnose yourself or use Google and easy access to drugs via the internet to replace a doctor who not only has scientific knowledge of these drugs but also knows your medical history.

Remember my patient with autism, Dominick? During his second visit, he and his mother told me that he was experiencing hunger and cravings, and so I prescribed a drug to help get those cravings under control. By his next visit, he was no longer struggling with feeling hungry, which made it easier for him to stay on track and lose thirty pounds.

There is one other thing I should mention about anti-obesity medications; among the over-the-counter selections available is a low-dosage, fat absorption inhibitor (a higher dosage is available as a prescription). But I never prescribe it, nor do I recommend it. First, it has some pretty nasty side effects (hint: wearing white or light-colored pants would not be wise while taking this drug because poor bowel control and dark, oily stools can result). Most importantly, though, the drug works by blocking the absorption of fat into the body, which goes against the entire premise of the No Guesswork Plan and what science has shown to be true about the benefits of a high-fat, low-carb diet.

With a BMI of nearly 57, Bill would have qualified for a prescription as well as bariatric surgery, but he wanted to try the No Guesswork Plan first without the medication or surgery. Once he started the plan, Bill just kept going with no stalls or stops. The two of us never even got around to discussing the surgical options. For many patients like Bill, surgery is indeed a viable option. If they have tried to lose weight for at least three months with no success, and they have a BMI of 40 or higher, they automatically meet the criteria to have a surgical procedure. I've discussed those procedures—the Lap Band, gastric sleeve, or gastric bypass (known scientifically as Roux-en-Y)—and the effectiveness of each of them in a previous chapter. Patients also can qualify if they have a BMI of 35 or more with an associated health condition, like type 2 diabetes or high blood pressure. As I mentioned in the earlier chapter, the sleeve and gastric bypass tend to be more successful because of their effect on ghrelin and the gastric bypass also has effects on the satiating gut hormones. The sleeve and gastric bypass cut out about 80 percent of the stomach, which means that it also cuts out about 80 percent of the ghrelin that lives in the stomach.

Interestingly, the sleeve was developed as a weight loss option by accident. Initially, it was used as a temporary measure for those whose obesity was so severe that they were a high surgical risk. They were not yet healthy enough to undergo the extensive surgery required for the gastric bypass (moving the small intestines closer to the stomach), so the sleeve was used in the early days as a first step to gastric bypass. The procedure was intended to assist in weight loss and give patients enough time to lose the weight, get healthier, and eventually undergo the full procedure. But a curious thing happened: some patients didn't return for the remaining surgery. Yet they kept losing weight and reached a satisfactory goal without a full gastric bypass. So the sleeve became a bona fide, less invasive surgical option.

A temporary fourth option—balloon-like devices that occupy space in the stomach—now can be used to help patients get to a healthier weight. They also can be used as a bridge for patients who must lose weight before they can be considered for weight-loss surgery. The FDA has approved these balloon-like space occupiers, which can be placed endoscopically in the stomach (two are placed endoscopically; one is actually swallowed by the patient) to help them feel full and lose weight. But the devices must be removed after six months.

Another FDA-approved device removes food from the stomach, and many other procedures are in the pipeline. Today, gastric bypass is still the most effective surgical procedure for weight loss because it eliminates 80 percent of the ghrelin that lives in the stomach and exposes the gut hormones to food sooner (since the small intestine is moved closer to the stomach), so a patient feels satiated and full quicker.

Making Low-Carb a Lifestyle

Fortunately for Bill, he learned to use food as his medicine, using protein and healthy fats to keep himself from getting hungry. His focus and determination were exemplary, and he remains the patient who has registered the biggest weight loss in my program. What impresses me even more than his weight loss is that Bill has managed to keep it off. Low-carb eating and exercise have become a lifestyle for him. We will discuss in the next chapter why exercise plays a greater role in maintaining weight than in weight loss. Through his exercise regimen, Bill has added more muscle to his frame, which increased the number on the scale a bit (muscle weighs more than fat), but he keeps his weight to around 240 pounds. That is the whole point of this program: I want to help you change your lifestyle so that you not only will lose weight but more importantly, keep it off for the rest of your life.

So, specifically, *how* did Bill do it?

The first major change that Bill made was to begin using a popular food tracking app to monitor his carbs (the NGW app is now available for even easier tracking). Tracking daily was a huge reality check for Bill. He learned very early that his perception of what he was eating and what he was actually eating were two totally different things. But the tracker helped him to plan and make better choices because it pushed him to think about how to get the "biggest bang for his buck," or which foods he could put together to allow himself large portions without going over his allotted carbs. For example, when he went to his favorite lunch spot, Subway, he began ordering a double chicken chopped salad instead of a sandwich and chips. Dinner mostly consisted of a double portion of meat and leafy green veggies. As mentioned earlier, he often broke dinner into three courses—salad, soup, meat, and veggies—and would get up from the table after each course to go get the next one. That automatically forced him to eat slower (remember it takes your brain about twenty minutes to realize you are full and your stomach is stretched to capacity), and by loading up on proteins and fat, quantity was rarely an issue.

Getting up between courses can help with weight loss, and food order can be important, too. A study done by Dr. Louis Aronne and some of his colleagues showed that the order in which you eat your food matters. If participants in the study ate protein first, followed by veggies and fat and then carbohydrates, their blood sugar and insulin levels were lower than if they ate carbohydrates first.

For Bill, it was really important to *feel* full, and so he kept mixing and matching food combinations to get to that point. In the beginning, he replaced the pasta, breads, and sweets in his diet with hearty proteins—grilled chicken, steak, hamburger, and other proteins and fats, none of which felt or tasted like traditional diet food. Then he made a big production of preparing his salads, washing, chopping, and mixing his own fresh vegetables and meats. He discovered some low-carb shirataki noodles, packaged in water, which he used for soups and stir-fry meals. He says he didn't miss his old lifestyle much because he never felt like he was missing out on things or that he was even on a diet. He kept a stash of protein bars handy for snacks.

Adding Exercise

For about the first six months, Bill was in no shape to join a gym. Concerned that he might hurt himself, I didn't even encourage it at first. I talked to him about Non-Exercise Activity Thermogenesis (NEAT), and he began squeezing in about 25 minutes of walking a day. He walked a little near home before work and got up from his desk at work to take a 15-minute walk around the office, the same time he would've taken for a coffee break. And one day it just occurred to him, instead of driving to the Subway for lunch, why not just walk there? From then on he and a co-worker walked there every day instead of driving. When he drove his car, he parked farther away than he normally would. He found he had less time to obsess about food, and he actually started to enjoy walking. So he gradually increased his steps.

For the first several months, Bill walked exclusively, eventually getting to a high of 25,000 steps per day. After about six months, he had lost enough weight and felt comfortable enough to join a gym, where he began working out with a trainer. His trainer started him on an exercise regimen using aqua kinetics, which is basically weight resistance training in the pool. The sessions lasted about an hour three days a week. The exercises focused on aerobics, like running in place and muscle building. Working out in the pool took the pressure off his knees and enabled him to exercise without hurting himself. In addition to the aqua kinetics, Bill also continued to walk a minimum of 15,000 steps a day. He reminded himself constantly that he was on a purposeful journey, which helped to keep him motivated to succeed.

After six months, Bill's trainer transitioned him into the gym. By then, Bill had regained some mobility, and he began working out in the gym at least five times a week— a regimen that is still a huge part of his life. He slowly scaled back his pool workout and got three or four different aerobic/resistance training programs from his trainer to mix up his routines a bit. What Bill began to realize is how often he had used food to fill the empty spaces in his life. When he was bored, he ate. When he felt down, he ate. And when he traveled with his job, he always looked for the best restaurants. Bill knew he had to address that within himself, so when he felt those urges to eat, he often would get up and take a walk. If he couldn't walk, he would snack on protein. And instead of looking for the best restaurants, he made a sport of looking for the best parks, and would then venture to one of those parks for a hike. One of his frequent travel spots was Portland, Oregon, where the food is pretty amazing, and food trucks are popular. But Bill also discovered that Portland, where a buddy from college lived, has 880 acres of amazing parks. In years past, the two friends often searched for good places to eat when Bill visited, but they transitioned from their food adventures to hiking adventures. During a college reunion, Bill and the same friend even broke away from the group and hiked Mount Greylock in Massachusetts while their classmates were eating and drinking. This was the same Bill who in the beginning walked no more than 1,000 steps a day. By the time he reached his goal, Bill was averaging 15,000 to 20,000 steps a day on a regular basis.

Bill's mindset change was about as dramatic as his physical change. He learned that he didn't lose anything, but he gained so much. He got his life back. This is the key, and this is what you should realize and focus on: you are not giving up anything, nor did you lose anything. In fact you gained so much. Bill really did get his life back. Among the many positive things I noticed about Bill was that he never missed a check-in with me. He weighed in, and we discussed his triumphs, challenges, and setbacks. The sessions were therapeutic, empowering Bill to open up and talk about whatever he wanted and to refuel for the next two weeks. The visits didn't only empower Bill; they also empowered me. I'd never gone on the journey Bill was on, but my job is to help people who are on that same journey. So I often asked

Bill questions to learn what the journey was like and then shared with other patients the information I got from his answers. Thanks to Bill, many of my other patients had some idea of what to expect. The meetings also provided some accountability. Although virtually everyone loses weight in my program, undoubtedly there are bumps in the road, causing many of them to stall. Bill and maybe one or two others were the only patients of mine who had lost weight EVERY time they came in for their appointment. It's a testament to Bill's dedication and diligence.

"Doc, your program works," Bill often said to me. It may seem self-evident, but if you do the program, you will lose weight. And if you don't follow the program, you'll have a harder time losing weight. When patients say, "Doc, my weight loss stalled," I work with them to figure out what the issues are, but in the end it turns out they just weren't truly following the program. There are either hidden carbs, or they are not tracking or not planning, or they are not making it to their appointment every two weeks. Every time I have such a conversation, I think back to Bill. He consistently tracked, planned, and made it to every weigh-in. And guess what? He lost weight and made it to his goal weight. I tried to figure out what motivated him to do the program exactly the way it was designed, so I could encourage others to do the same. And I realized, the weigh-ins were crucial for Bill. They provided accountability. Accountability is important. So, for each of you who decide to take this journey, you have to build in a system of accountability and support, perhaps with your family doctor and/or my online support group. Some of the people in the group have been on the journey a bit longer and can help to encourage and support you.

The other thing that helps put things in perspective is my Hunt Motivational Scale (HMS). It gives you a score of how well you're doing. If you score high you will do well and lose weight. If you score low you won't do as well and you likely won't lose weight as predicted. If you find you are not doing well, focus on the areas where your score is low to improve that area and overall score. Use the HMS as often as you like to help keep you focused and on track (the HMS is at the end of **Chapter Five**).

Bill's journey is ongoing. After losing so much weight, Bill had to have three surgeries to remove excess skin. Each intricate surgery lasted about six hours. At first, Bill was apprehensive about the scars, but he says his mind had to evolve on that issue, as well. He realized he had to stop defining success by the perfect images he saw in magazines and on the television screen; otherwise, it would have been easy to give up. Now, Bill's goal is to stay the course. "The wolf is always at the door," he says, reminding himself not to let his guard down.

These days, Bill has more reason than ever to stay on track. About two years after he started his journey with me, Bill married the love of his life, and they now have a set of beautiful twins. Bill is so grateful that he changed his life because he is now able to be fully engaged with his wife and children, fully engaged in life.

CHAPTER 10
PHASE THREE—Maintenance

Congratulations! You've reached your goal weight. Now you begin Phase Three—Maintenance. If you've made it this far, this should be a proud moment for you. If not, just keep going. You can do it! Reaching the Maintenance Phase is a major accomplishment, like finally landing a plane that has been in the air for months. That's really what Phase One and Phase Two were all about: preparing you for landing in Maintenance. You probably experienced a bit of turbulence along the way, but hopefully you reached a cruising altitude, a space where the journey felt smooth and comfortable. You are surely feeling better, looking better, and living a healthier lifestyle. You have changed your life. Take a moment to reflect on how far you've come, as well as the commitment and discipline it took to get here. Bask in your success! In my clinic, I give patients who reach this milestone a certificate and pin to recognize their achievement (a copy of the certificate is on the next page for you when you reach your goal. Congratulations! Just print it out at www.noguesswork.com, complete it and display proudly). It's okay to reward yourself, as long as you don't fall back into the old habit of using the wrong foods to celebrate. Treat yourself to a fun adventure. Buy something you've been eyeing for a while. Go dancing. Or just give yourself a well-deserved pat on the back. You deserve to feel amazing!

NGW

NO GUESSWORK CERTIFICATE OF ACHIEVEMENT

IS AWARDED TO

____

For Completion of Phase 2 and getting to your goal weight.
Now you are officially in Maintenance!
Weight Management Program

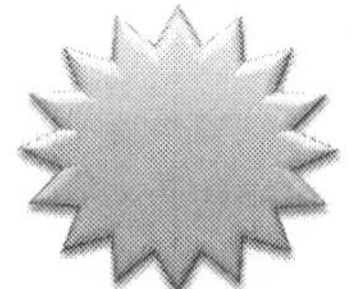

RAMECK HUNT

RAMECK HUNT, MD, FACP

Now that you are in Maintenance I want you to fill out the Hunt Motivational Scale (HMS) for Maintenance (on the next page). Just like the HMS you filled out for active weight loss, this HMS will give you a score and help keep you on track. The higher your score, the better you will be in Maintenance. So if your score is low, focus on the area where your score is low and improve it, so you can make sure you maintain your weight loss.

HUNT MOTIVATIONAL SCALE
MAINTENANCE

PATIENT NAME: ______________________________

DOB:____________________ Date:________________

IN THE PAST 2 WEEKS, HOW WELL HAVE YOU DONE THE FOLLOWING:

1. Do you do planned physical activity on a daily basis (i.e. walking, heavy gardening, going to the gym, etc)?
   0 (never) 1 (inconsistently) 2 (consistently)*

2. Do you eat on a regular schedule daily?
   0 (never) 1 (inconsistently) 2 (consistently)

3. Are you tracking your food?
   0 (never) 1 (inconsistently) 2 (consistently)

4. Are you at your maintenance carb (or calorie) goal?
   0 (never) 1 (inconsistently) 4 (consistently)

5. Do you weigh yourself at least once per week?
   (never) 1 (inconsistently) 2 (consistently)

6. Do you limit yourself to less than 1-hour worth of screen time after you get off work (tv, internet, etc)?
   (never) 1 (inconsistently) 2 (consistently)

7. Based off the trigger foods that we have identified, have you been able to avoid your identified trigger foods?
   0 (never) 1 (inconsistently) 2 (consistently)

Score: ________
11-16 (predicts you will continue to do well)
7-10 (Average score. Predicts you may or may not continue to maintain your weight. Work to get your number in the 10-12 range)
4-6 (Below average. Predicts you may not do well in maintenance. We have to figure out how to get your number higher. Work to get your number in the 10-12 range)
0-3 (This is dangerous. Predicts you will likely regain weight. We have to come up with a plan to stabilize you in maintenance)

*consistently is defined as 80%-90% of the times (4 out of 5 times)

If you are not yet at your goal weight, don't get so frustrated about the time it's taking you to get there that you forget to celebrate the weight loss you've accomplished already. A weight loss of at least 10 percent of your body weight puts you farther ahead in the game than most people. You are at a healthier weight, and you, too, should be proud. Sometimes, though, pride is not at all what my patients feel when they aren't yet where they want to be after a certain amount of time. This reminds me of one particular patient named Cara.

Cara's goal was to lose 100 pounds. She did really well in the beginning, completing Phase One and losing 10 percent of her body weight in a little over three months. She kept going, and by the end of a year she was down 50 pounds. But around the holidays at the end of the first year, life hit her with a huge blow, the death of her mother. As Cara grieved, her weight loss slowed, and it just seemed difficult for her to get going again at the same pace. Fortunately, she didn't fall back into her old habit of overdosing on carbs, but the discipline that had helped her succeed in the beginning slipped. She wasn't tracking, so she couldn't be exactly sure whether she was staying under her carb number.

On one of Cara's visits, she expressed frustration that she had not yet reached her goal weight. By this point, she had been in the program for about two years and hadn't lost any more weight of significance since that initial 50 pounds. She was frustrated that with everything else going on in her life, she seemed stuck at that 50-pound mark. I had to remind Cara (and remind myself), that she'd lost 50 pounds! And that's not too shabby. But more importantly I had to point out to her that she'd been able to maintain her lower weight, keeping that 50 pounds off for more than two years! Sure, we'd been doing this for a while, and she wasn't quite where she wanted to be yet. But she was much healthier than when she was 50 pounds heavier, and that, in itself, is a huge achievement. Upwards of 90 percent of people who lose that much weight gain it right back. So I remind my patients, like I reminded Cara, that they (and perhaps you, my friend) are in a unique club—part of the 10 percent of people who are succeeding in keeping the weight off. Don't knock yourself if it's taking more time than you expected to get to your final goal weight.

Now, if you are at your goal weight, let's talk about this sobering reality: your journey is not yet complete. In fact, this part (keeping the weight off) will be the longest leg of all. As I've stressed many times, my No Guesswork program is not just another diet. It is a lifestyle. You have learned how to eat and live healthier. To maintain the goal you have reached, you have to keep doing what you did to get here (with a few adjustments that I will discuss in a bit).

As noted, it's common for people who lose at least 10 percent of their body weight to regain. We've seen it many times—friends or family members go on a fad diet, lose a significant amount of weight, and almost as soon as the diet ends, the weight gain begins. Up next, we'll look at the science behind it.

Going to Extremes

A study of fourteen contestants who participated in the once wildly popular televised weight loss show, *The Biggest Loser*, provides some insight into why keeping the weight off is so tough. Researchers at the National Institutes of Health in Bethesda, Maryland, studied contestants who participated in Season Eight of the show, which aired in 2009. Thousands of viewers across the globe tuned in each week to watch the contestants, who started at an average of 328 pounds, follow a brutal workout regimen and overcome fat-burning and discipline challenges in a battle for the title of

"The Biggest Loser." With the world watching, the desperate contestants shared in detail their battles with weight, competed in various workout challenges, and at the end of each episode stepped onto the scale to reveal how much weight they had lost. Over the season, they dropped to an astonishing average of 200 pounds. But when researchers measured the fourteen contestants six years later, all but one of them had regained the bulk of the weight, if not all of it; four were even heavier than before the show.

The winner of Season Eight, Danny Cahill, lost more than half of his body weight, dropping from 430 pounds to 191 by the show's finale. His 239-pound weight loss was a greater percentage of weight loss than any other male contestant had accomplished in the history of the show. On the night of his victory, he was understandably jubilant: "I've got my life back," he proclaimed. But when researchers weighed and measured Cahill six years later, he had regained 100 pounds, according to a *New York Times* magazine story about the NIH study. The study showed that the average weight of the six men and eight women who participated had gone back up to 290 pounds. The study also revealed the contestants' metabolism had slowed dramatically, showing they were burning far fewer calories daily after losing the weight than before appearing on the show.

We in the medical profession expect your rate of metabolism to decrease when you lose weight because you don't need as much energy to fuel a smaller body (much like a smaller house doesn't need as much heat as a larger house would), but these contestant's metabolism decreased even more than one would predict (15 percent more than was predicted!). And even after they regained the weight, their metabolism still did not return to normal. Why didn't it return to normal? Let's take a look at the process.

When a person's metabolism slows down, he or she has to eat fewer calories to keep from gaining weight. But six years after being crowned The Biggest Loser, Cahill's metabolism had slowed so much that he had to consume 800 fewer calories per day than a typical man his size, 295 pounds, just to stay at that weight. Most of the other contestants had to eat an average of 500 fewer calories than a person of their size to avoid gaining weight.

A slowed metabolism is one of the ways the body fights to get back to what it perceives as your baseline/normal weight, or—as I've described earlier—your set point. This is a part of what is called "metabolic adaptation," which we will discuss in more detail later in this chapter. But *The Biggest Loser* contestants' metabolism slowed to an extreme degree. Why? The data appears to show that the extraordinary measures the contestants took to lose the weight (grueling, all-day workouts and significant calorie reductions in their meals) influenced the dramatic slowdown of their metabolism. It was an extreme instance of metabolic adaptation. Their bodies overcompensated, making some of them gain back even more weight than when they started. It was the body's outsize response to the exaggerated way they lost weight.

When the Body Fights Back

So how does your body fight you to get back to your set point? What happens is complex and involves multiple factors, but I will try to simplify it here. When you lose weight, your body will try to get you back to what it perceives as normal by making you hungrier and making you crave more. A study done by Dr. Michael Rosenbaum and other researchers showed that participants had a higher desire for a particular food when they lost 10 percent of their body weight than before they lost weight. This was confirmed by tests showing that areas of the brain that are responsible for cravings lit up more after the participants lost weight than when they were at their baseline weight. This means their cravings were stronger. The study also showed that it took more food for that same person to feel satisfied after they lost 10 percent of their body weight. This is caused by the gut hormones that I discussed earlier in the book—the hunger/craving hormone (ghrelin, aka the Hunger Gremlin) and the many satiating hormones (GLP-1, PYY, etc.). And then your body does a number of things to decrease your metabolism, including making your muscles work more efficiently to conserve energy and decreasing your adrenaline.

As I mentioned earlier in this book, your body can't make you grab a Big Mac, but it can increase the hunger hormone and decrease the satiating hormone so that you feel hungrier, and your cravings are so strong that you need and want more food to feel satisfied. And then on top of that, your body slows down the rate in which you burn off those calories and fat. The net effect is that you eat more and burn less energy until your body gets you back to what it considers your normal/baseline weight. Once you get back to that point, your body settles down again. Your hormones normalize, and your metabolism usually goes back to normal.

The good news is that most people who lose weight don't necessarily suffer the drastic metabolism slowdown that *The Biggest Loser* contestants experienced after the show. Other research has shown that while the metabolism indeed slows for most people who lose weight, it only slows a bit, and the slowdown may occur for just a short while. A 2018 study by Dr. David Ludwig of Harvard University and several of his colleagues shows that you can preserve your metabolism if you eat a low-carb diet that is high in fat and moderately high in protein (a well-formulated low-carb diet). So that's one of the reasons why my program is formulated as such.

Medication: There if You Need It

The body routinely tries to protect itself, specifically its fat mass. It's an instinctual survival mechanism. Sometimes, this may mean that medication is needed to block the process of the body trying to get you to regain weight. If you're struggling with hunger and cravings after you lose weight, you may feel defeated. But it's not all gloom and doom, because doctors who treat obesity, like me, understand more about what is happening. In the past, we really didn't understand this phenomenon and just blamed the patient. They just needed more discipline, we told them. These days, though, because we understand the problem, we know how to combat it. We can do this first with diet (a low-carb diet with healthy fat and protein) and if needed, the new medications that block the body's efforts to regain weight.

Not only are medications helpful to some people throughout their weight loss journey, they also may be useful to help keep them in maintenance. One small study of fifty adults with overweight and obesity had them lose weight on a meal replacement diet. Researchers measured the participants' gut hormones at baseline (the beginning of the study), at 10 weeks, and again at 62 weeks. At the one-year mark, the gut hormone levels persisted in an imbalance that favored weight gain. That study shows that the body will continue trying to pull you back to what it perceives as normal, even a year later.

Some patients tell me they don't want to take medications, whether it's for their blood pressure, diabetes, cholesterol, or even to get to a healthier weight. "Doc, give me a few more months to work on this myself," they say. And I always use my umbrella analogy. If it's raining, you would use an umbrella to protect you from the rain, right? And then, when the rain stops, you put the umbrella away. Same with your health. While you work on making lifestyle changes, wouldn't it be a good idea to protect yourself from the rain (i.e. diabetes, obesity, etc.)? And then when you've made those lifestyle changes and the rain stops (i.e. your diabetes or weight is controlled), we put the umbrella away (i.e. stop the medicine). When I put it like that, my patients tend to understand better. Who wouldn't want to be protected until it stops raining? The same goes for your health. If you are trying lifestyle changes for your diabetes, cholesterol, high blood pressure, or even your weight, and the lifestyle changes you are making have not yet controlled those things, don't be afraid to put up an umbrella to protect you from the rain in the meantime. And when it stops raining and things are under control, you can always put the umbrella away.

Exercise

Research has helped us in the medical community understand what happens to our bodies when we lose weight and why it happens. As a result, we also have a better understanding of what to do to counteract those negative effects. Remember when I told you that to lose weight, your diet (what you put in your mouth) was more important than exercise at a ratio of about 80 percent to 20 percent? In the Maintenance Phase, diet and exercise are equally important, 50/50. To overcome the decrease in your metabolism, you have to purposefully increase your physical activity, either by increasing your exercise regimen, increasing your NEAT (Non-Exercise Activity Thermogenesis), or better yet, by increasing both to compensate for the decrease in metabolism.

I want you to understand in detail just what you need to do to keep the weight off. But first, let's get some basics out of the way. You need to get good sleep at night, at least six hours (preferably seven to eight hours). You also need stress management (exercise, meditation, yoga, etc.). Without those things, your hormones get out of whack, and you are tempted to overeat. Got it? Now for the strategy. Let's start with physical activity and recap how your metabolism works.

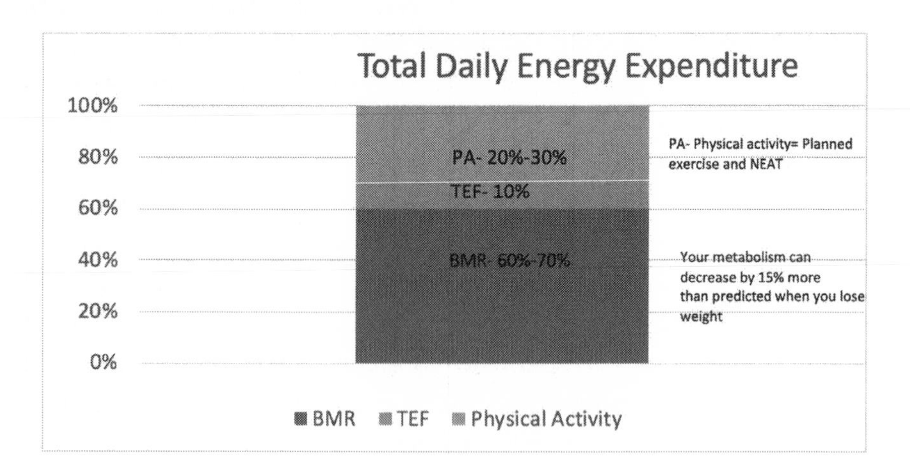

On a daily basis, our metabolism makes up for about 60-70 percent of the energy we expend. The energy you expend on digestion is about 10 percent, and the rest of the energy we expend (20-30 percent) is made up of our physical activity (exercise and NEAT).

As I mentioned, your body can decrease your basal metabolism by about 15 percent more than predicted in an effort to get you to regain the weight you lost. There's no way to prevent this; you have very little control over your BMR (Basal Metabolic Rate), the baseline energy your body burns before any physical activity and TEF (Thermogenic Effects of Food, the energy you spend to digest food).

There may be some things you can do to offset the decrease in metabolism, however, such as an increase in your physical activity. That is the only factor you can really control. To make up for the drop in metabolism, you would need to increase in your physical activity by more than that 15 percent. The easiest way to do that is to focus on your NEAT, the things you do to expend energy that are not part of a workout routine. In other words, try to be more mobile and active during your normal daily activities. The other thing that may help maintain your metabolism, based off a study done by

Dr. Ludwig, is to eat a well formulated low-carb diet (high fat, moderate protein and low-carb).

A consistent increase in NEAT is more reliable than planned exercising, in my opinion (although planned exercise is vitally important, as well). How many times did you plan to exercise in the morning or after work, and then life got in the way? Therefore, I encourage you to examine the things you do every day and figure out how to expend more energy doing them. I want you to think about how you can change your lifestyle regarding NEAT. When you park your vehicle at work or at the mall, can you park farther away from the entrance so that you have to walk a longer distance? Can you take the stairs, instead of the elevator, at all times? Can you walk to your favorite lunch spot? When you need to talk to a co-worker, can you walk to her office, instead of picking up the phone? For most people, the goal should be to take *greater* than 10,000 steps per day. If you have a medical condition that prevents you from taking that many steps (like severe arthritis), that's okay. You can focus on moving your upper body more.

I developed another term that I call SEAT, which stands for Small Exercise Activity Thermogenesis, exercises that you do while sitting at work or home. That includes leg raises, arm lunges, using your desk or wall for push-ups, etc. You can find some examples of SEAT exercises on the No Guesswork website and/or app. But feel free to come up with your own SEAT exercises. Just be safe. Make sure your desk and chair are stable enough to do the exercises. If you have a rolling seat, make sure you lock it.

Making up that 15 percent decrease in BMR is critical to maintaining weight loss. Your increased physical activity has to be consistent. So maximizing your NEAT and SEAT is key. Make sure you are doing everything you can to burn energy during your normal activities.

Ideally, a Maintenance plan includes NEAT, SEAT, *and* planned exercise. For good health, the American College of Sports Medicine (ACMS) recommends 150 minutes per week, or 30 minutes of moderate exercise five days per week, for the average person. If you have a gym membership, that's great. Schedule an appointment to go to the gym, as you would schedule an important appointment at work. If you can't afford to go to the gym or just don't like working out in a gym, set a time to take a brisk walk in your neighborhood before or after work every day. Commitment is key. There will never be a perfect time, so you have to make the time to exercise, like you make the time to do the other things in your life that are important to you.

Maintenance Strategies

So, as discussed, once you lose the weight, you may get strong cravings and perhaps feel hungrier at times than you did before you lost weight. It's inevitable. The foods you are craving may be even more desirable than they were at your baseline weight, and it likely will take more to make you feel more satisfied (particularly on a low-calorie, higher-carb diet). As I've mentioned, some studies suggest that a consistent low-carb, high-fat diet may prevent that from happening. Let this be a motivation to continue tracking your food, planning your low-carb, high-fat meals, and/or meal prepping to help you maintain control and stay on track.

You can win the battle against hunger and cravings with this strategy: Use protein as a medicine to decrease those feelings. Protein is the strongest macronutrient that can suppress ghrelin. So keep high-protein snacks available (a hardboiled egg, single-serve peanut butter pack, string cheese, meat stick/jerky, protein shake, 100-calorie pack of almonds, etc.). Also, eat on a schedule to keep ghrelin suppressed around the clock. Consider eating a pre-meal protein snack. If such strategies worked when you were in Phases One and Two, continue them. And continue to keep your carbs low. By now, you know that eating an excess of carbs will increase insulin, promote fat storage, and light up your craving center (your limbic system) to make you crave more carbs. Plus, in just three to four hours, you will feel hungry again, particularly if you've indulged in sugar and refined carbohydrates, and the cycle keeps repeating itself. So, stick to the principle of eating primarily proteins/healthy fats and green veggies.

In the Maintenance Phase you can increase your intake of carbs slightly. You even get a new carb number, called your Weight Maintenance Carb Number (WMCN). Before we go into detail on this, let me reiterate the basics about your carb numbers. Your Weight Loss Carb Number (WLCN) is based on your personal threshold—the maximum number of carbs you can eat and lose weight. If you stay beneath that threshold, you will lose weight. If you go above that threshold, the weight loss will stop. You shouldn't gain weight if you stay within a certain range above that threshold, but you won't lose weight either. I call this range in which your weight remains stable the buffer zone. However, if you continue to increase your carbs and go outside of that range, you will begin to gain weight. That top number, the number you need to stay below to avoid gaining weight, is your Weight Maintenance Carb Number (WMCN). For example, if your Weight Loss Carb Number is 50, once you go above 50 your weight loss shuts off, but you shouldn't gain weight immediately; you will stay in the buffer zone. Let's say that you notice you start gaining weight when you exceed an average of 60 grams of carbs a week. In that case, your buffer zone is an average from 50 to 60 grams of carbs per week. So, your actual Weight Maintenance Carb Number is 60 (the number you need to stay below to avoid weight gain, in other words, your weight *gain* carb number). Got it? See the graph below, which demonstrates this point.

WEIGHT LOSS, BUFFER ZONE AND WEIGHT MAINTENANCE CARB NUMBERS

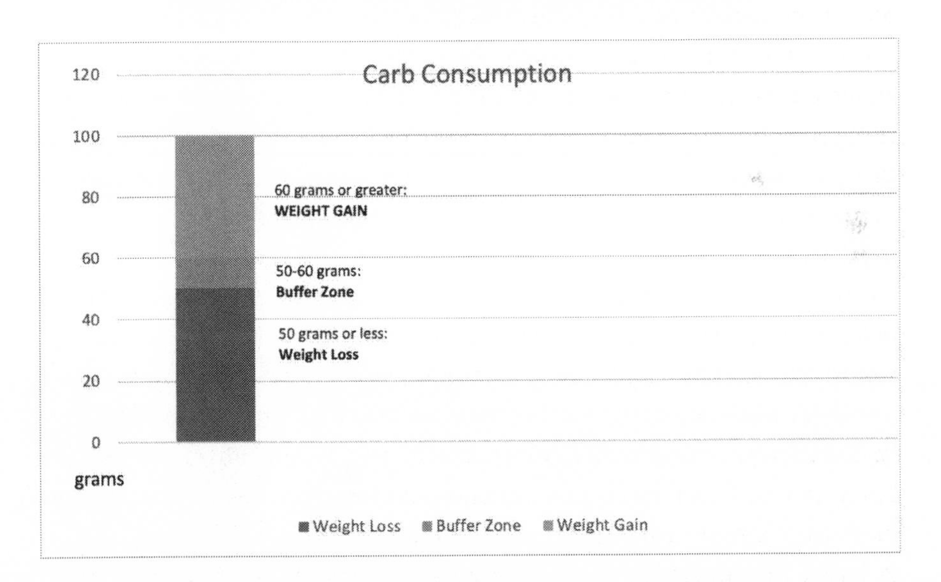

For the average person, your Weight Maintenance Carb Number will be about 20 percent higher than your Weight Loss Carb Number (WLCN). For example, if your Weight Loss Carb Number was 50 grams, you would take 20 percent of 50, which is 10 grams, and add it to 50, giving you a Weight Maintenance Carb Number of 60. To confirm that number, try it out for two weeks. If your weight doesn't change, you can stay there. Your threshold may be even a little higher, so if you want to test it, you can add an additional 5 grams of carbs every two weeks until you get to a point where you start gaining. If that happens, just ratchet the number down again by 5 carbs each week until your weight stabilizes, and you most likely have found your exact maintenance number.

If you noticed weight gain right away in your first weigh-in after increasing your Weight Loss Carb Number by 20 percent, just drop that number by 5 carbs the next week and, if needed, repeat until your weight stabilizes. Remember, this is a process, but once you know your Weight Maintenance Carb Number, you know what it will take to maintain your same weight.

Mediterranean Eating

So now that you know your Weight Loss Carb Number (WLCN) and you've found your weight maintenance carb number (WMCN), you are all set! You can use those two numbers to navigate the rest of your life. Congratulations!

Even though you are now starting to add a few more carbs back into your diet, don't go overboard. Keep in mind that most, if not all, of the carbs you add should come from fiber. You've made a lifestyle change, and this is not a return to the same unhealthy stuff you used to eat. Continue to avoid sugary foods and refined carbohydrates, such as white flour products, pastries, pastas, and foods that have been processed and stripped of their nutritional value. The goal during the Maintenance Phase, what I like to call *Your Forever Phase,* is to eat a low-carb Mediterranean Diet, a heart-healthy meal plan that consists primarily of fresh vegetables, low-carb fruits (blueberries, strawberries, etc.), legumes (beans, peas, lentils), whole grains, fish, poultry, nuts, olive oil, and even red wine. These are the kinds of carbs that you can begin to add to your meals in moderation.

The Mediterranean Diet is based on the traditional foods of African and European countries that border the Mediterranean Sea (Greece, Italy, France, Morocco, Turkey, Egypt, Libya, Algeria, Tunisia and Spain), whose people tended to live longer and suffer fewer instances of heart disease and cancer than people of the United States. Studies have shown the Mediterranean Diet is the best for long-term, good heart health. Two more interesting facts about the Mediterranean Diet. First, there is something called the French paradox. France is one of the Mediterranean countries, and even though the French consume high amounts of saturated fats, they had fewer deaths from heart disease than the UK or the United States. One thought was that the French are protected from heart disease because of all the red wine that they drink, but studies showed that this was not likely the case since they didn't or couldn't drink nearly enough red wine to see any significant beneficial effects. The real reason is likely multifactorial, but it's clear that the French ate more saturated fats (as well as more monounsaturated and polyunsaturated fats) yet have less heart disease.

As I mentioned in earlier chapters, saturated fats have not been definitely shown to cause heart disease. However, sugar and refined carbohydrates have been shown to be associated with heart disease. This was demonstrated in a re-analysis of data from fourteen of the countries we discussed in Chapter 2, revealing a direct correlation between sugar intake and death.

Another thing about the French was that they ate more whole foods. And guess what they ate less of? Processed and ultra-processed foods full of sugars and refined carbohydrates (sound familiar?). In general, those who eat a Mediterranean diet eat more fat (approximately 40%-60% or more), and this is the diet that has been shown to be the best diet for your heart based on multiple studies.

The second interesting fact about the Mediterranean diet is that the first person who has been credited for making the Mediterranean diet popular is none other than the anti-fat guru himself, Ancel Keys. His Seven Country Study is the first study that demonstrated the heart benefits of a Mediterranean diet. It was this study that showed Keys that total fat didn't increase heart disease, but the study did show an increase in heart disease with increasing saturated fats based off the countries he selected to be in the study (interestingly, he did not include France in this study or in his previous six country data that I mentioned earlier). Ultimately, Keys touted the high fat (mostly monounsaturated and polyunsaturated fats) Mediterranean diet as the best diet for heart health based on this study. So Keys abandoned his theory of total fat being the cause of heart disease and focused on saturated fats as being the culprit. Even though the French diet was a Mediterranean diet with high saturated fat, the Mediterranean diet Keys recommended (the same one that is recommended today), although high in total fat, was not high in saturated fat. Again, the bottom line is a well formulated low-carb Mediterranean diet is best for weight loss and heart health (and best for all the 6 S's I mentioned earlier in the book) based on the available evidence.

Normal Mediterranean Diet

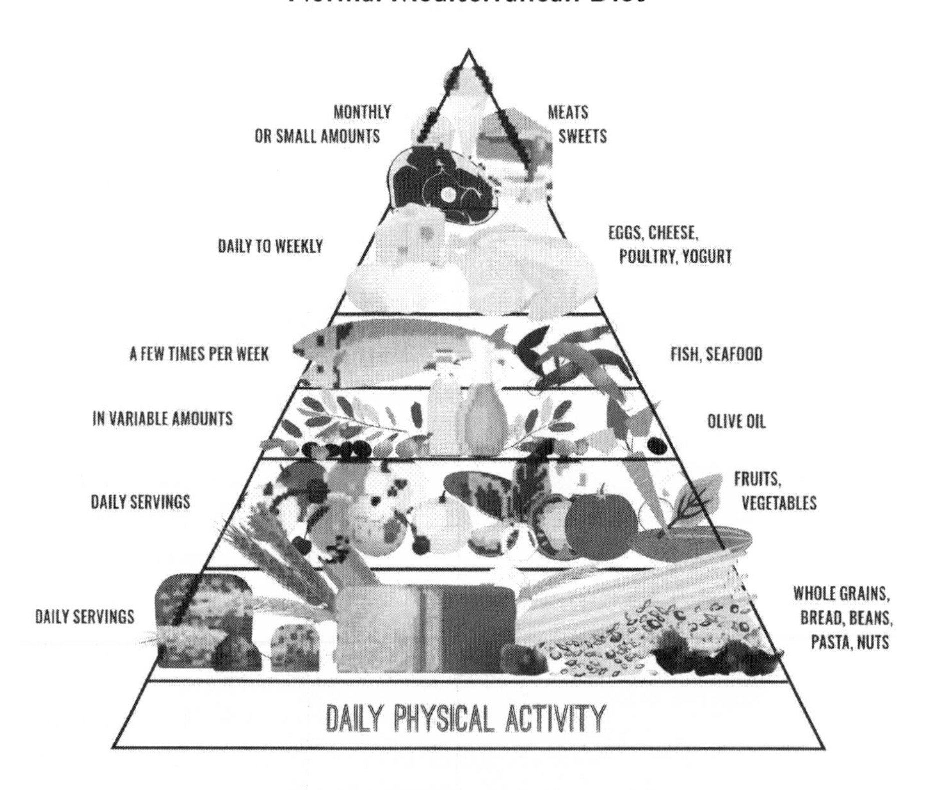

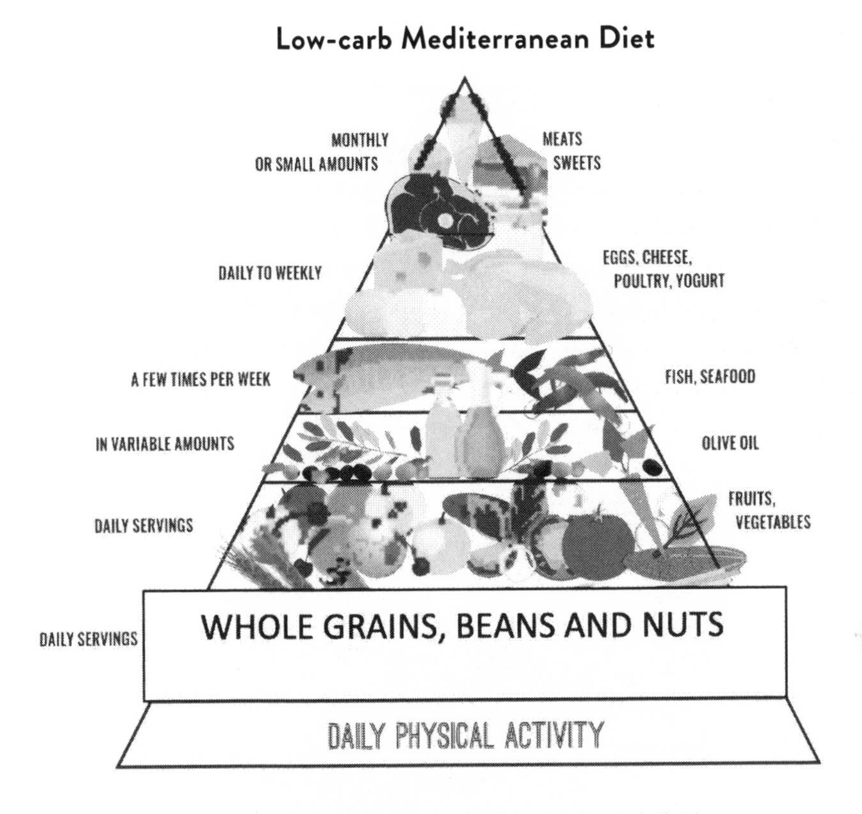

Low-carb MEDITERRANEAN DIET

That said, even though you can add back carbs (mostly in the form of fiber), you still have to stay below your Weight Maintenance Carb Number. If you are struggling to maintain your weight loss, you should see your doctor, or if possible, an obesity medicine specialist. These medical professionals can help you balance out the hormones that are trying to tip your body in favor of weight regain. If you start to gain unhealthy weight (fat instead of muscle), the doctor may ask you to consider taking an anti-obesity medication, even if you didn't need any medication throughout your weight loss phase. I mentioned in an earlier chapter that there are new prescription drugs on the market to help settle your hormones.

*****

One last thing, let's talk about weigh-ins. Once you get to your goal weight, you have to monitor your weight regularly. I recommend you continue to weigh yourself at least once a week, and I'd even encourage you to weigh yourself more than that. If your weight goes up by three pounds, take a look around you. What are you doing differently? "Nothing" is not an adequate response. Be honest with yourself. The odds are that if you gained a little weight, you exceeded your Weight Maintenance Carb Number. Check your tracker and make sure you have been below your WMCN on average. If not, return to your Weight *Loss* Carb Number to get those pounds off, and then remain diligent about staying below your Weight Maintenance Carb Number. Remember; this is your Forever Phase. If you were at your Weight Maintenance Carb Number when you gained weight, you may have to do some troubleshooting, like we discussed in the weight loss phase (look out for hidden carbs, make sure your physical activity is the same, etc. Also fill out the Hunt Motivational Scale to help you troubleshoot. Then focus on the areas where your score may be low). Once you figure out the issue, do the same as above, return to your WLCN until you get back to your Maintenance weight and then go back and live at your WMCN.

All along, be very diligent and consistent about tracking and, of course, keeping your carbs down. If you still find it difficult and/or you find that you are struggling with serious cravings and/or hunger, your body may be fighting you to get you back to your set point. In that case, I suggest you find an obesity medicine specialist to help.

So, to recap: Yes, your body will fight for years to get you back to your baseline weight. But YOU can combat that by increasing your NEAT (the energy you expend doing every day activities) and/or SEAT (small exercises that you do while seated at your desk or on the sofa) and adding a consistent exercise regimen to your daily routine. You should also use protein and healthy fats to fight off the strong cravings and hunger you may feel. But you must continue to track and plan. That is the responsibility you have to be accountable to yourself. If you don't do it, stop there until you get that part right. It's just that important. Then, if you are still struggling to keep the weight off, find an obesity medicine specialist in your area. And don't panic if the doctor suggests medication to counteract what your body is doing to get you back to your baseline weight (Remember what I said about metabolic adaptation? We have to combat that).

Some of this news may seem disheartening. You may wonder, why did I work so hard to lose the weight if my own body will fight me to regain it? My response is simple: You are worth the fight! Because you know exactly what you're fighting, you know *how* to fight. And you CAN win! You've come too far to lose hope. Your health and your life are at stake. YOU are a winner!

Afterword

We covered a lot in this book, and you did it! You successfully achieved weight loss and have maintained a healthier weight. So, I want to take a moment to recap all the important points that you should remember.

IT'S ALL ABOUT YOUR NUMBER! #What'sYourCarbNumber

1. Find your Weight Loss Carb Number (WLCN). You do that by decreasing your carbs to less than 100 grams and try to get closer to 50 grams per day. Your starting target should be 75 grams per day and work from there. If you lose at least one to two pounds per week, average your weekly carb number; that average most likely is your Weight Loss Carb Number (WLCN). Then for the next two weeks stay below that number to confirm. If you continue to lose one to two pounds per week, then you know that this is your WLCN. (Refer to Chapter Five for details)
2. Continue to stay below your WLCN through Phases One and Two until you reach your goal weight.
3. Weight Maintenance Carb Number (WMCN)—once you get to your goal weight, it's time to find your Weight Maintenance Carb Number (WMCN). To get started, first estimate your Weight Maintenance Carb Number (WMCN) by taking 20 percent of your WLCN and adding it to your WLCN. So if your WLCN is 50 grams per day, then your estimated WMCN is 60 grams per day (20 percent of 50 is 10 and 50 + 10= 60). Try that number out, and if you maintain your weight over the next two weeks, then you have likely found your number. However, your threshold may be even a little higher, so if you want to test it, you can add an additional five grams

of carbs every two weeks until you get to a point where you start gaining. Whatever the number is when you start gaining weight, just decrease it by five grams, and that will be your absolute threshold to your Weight Maintenance Carb Number. For example, if you were increasing your WMCN by five grams every two weeks, and when you get to 70 grams of carbs per day, you gained one to two pounds, then return to 65 grams of carbs per day. If your weight stabilizes, then 65 grams of carbs is your WMCN. See above in Chapter 10 for details.

4. Physical activity—Even though 80 percent of weight loss is diet and 20 percent is physical activity, physical activity is still very important. And physical activity becomes even more important in the Maintenance phase. In fact, physical activity is 50 percent of weight maintenance. Planned exercise is important, but what's even more important is what's called NEAT (Non-exercise Activity Thermogenesis). If you exercise two to three times per week, that still would only amount to about two to three hours of a 168-hour week. That leaves another 165 hours in the week, and that's where NEAT (the activities that cause you to expend energy during the normal course of your day) comes in. You can maximize that 165 hours (minus sleep, of course) with NEAT (and SEAT-Small Exercise Activity Thermogenesis) by expanding your usual activities with changes, such as parking further away from the door, which causes you to walk further. Both NEAT/SEAT and planned exercise are very important, so you need to do both, but make sure to maximize your NEAT/SEAT and get whatever planned exercise you can.
5. Remember that your body has a set point, and it will work to get you back to what it perceives as normal. It does that by adjusting your gut hormones and decreasing your metabolism (this is called metabolic adaptation). But don't fret because knowledge is power, and as you learned in this book, there are ways to combat it.
6. Remember the mindset of change. This is a lifestyle change. Once you get to your goal, you are in your Forever Phase.
7. Finally, remember to stick to a well-formulated low-carb diet that is full of healthy fats and protein.

14-Day Meal Guide

You're busy. You have a full life and lots of people in it, but perhaps looking after loved ones has left you taking care of everyone but yourself. You've finally decided to change your life by changing what you eat, but putting together menu ideas that the entire family can enjoy is just one more thing on your already full plate. So we've done a little of the work for you.

In this section, you will find a 14-day meal plan with the estimated carbs for each item. Of course, the carb count will vary based on how you prepare your food and portion size, so always use your app (NGW, My Fitness Pal, or whatever you're using to track your food intake) to double check the carb count. This is especially important if you spice things up by adding sauces or yummy toppings, or any ingredients that may increase the amount of carbs. Go ahead and let your creativity flow with these menu ideas, but remember that if you add carbs in one item, you may need to make an adjustment elsewhere to even things out. Also, you may need to subtract some items (or may want to add more), depending on your personalized carb number.

This is not a diet plan! I repeat: You do not have to follow this menu guide exactly, or at all. But it's there if you need it, and you can replace items you don't like with something else, or mix and match foods that you think would work better together. Remember, you are in control of what you put in your mouth. These are just *suggestions* to help jumpstart your transition and make planning your meals a bit easier until putting together low-carb menu choices becomes second nature.

Many of the menu items in this section are so basic that you likely will not even need a recipe to cook them. However, thanks to Google (or whatever computer search engine you prefer), you don't have to stress if you need a guide to figure out just how much seasoning to put on that chicken breast. All of these recipes can be found online. I did include a basic recipe for Bulletproof coffee (as promised earlier in the book), as well as an easy-to-cook menu item, called chaffles, which have become extremely popular among people following a low-carb diet. They are basically low-carb mini-waffles, made with cheese, eggs, and almond flour, but you can add sweet or savory flavorings to make a dish that can replace not only high-carb waffles, but also English muffins, sandwich buns, pizza, and more!

Easy Bulletproof Coffee Recipe

(2 servings)

2 cups black coffee
2 tablespoons grass-fed butter
2 tablespoons coconut oil
2 teaspoons heavy cream

Brew two cups of coffee using freshly ground coffee beans (or your coffee of choice). In a large pitcher (or two separate cups) mix in butter, oil, and cream. Mix well. Serve coffee and enjoy.

Basic Chaffles

1 cup mozzarella cheese
1 egg
1 tablespoon almond flour
1 teaspoon baking powder
1 teaspoon vanilla flavor
Dash of cinnamon
(You will need a mini waffle-maker to make this recipe)

Set aside ¼ cup mozzarella cheese. Mix remaining ingredients together in a mixing bowl. Place mini-waffle maker on a plate to avoid a messy clean-up in case the mixture spills out of the sides. Plug in the waffle maker and spray it with oil. When the waffle maker is hot, sprinkle ¼ cup of cheese on the griddle. When the cheese is melted, spoon a thin layer of the mixture over the griddle, covering it. Close the top and allow the chaffle to cook about 4 minutes. When the chaffle is golden brown in color and crispy around the edges, remove it carefully. Add butter and your favorite low-carb syrup. This recipe makes about 4 mini-chaffles. Enjoy!

Pepperoni Pizza Chaffles

½ cup mozzarella cheese
1 large egg
1 tablespoon almond flour
1 teaspoon oregano
1 teaspoon garlic powder
1 teaspoon red pepper flakes
Pepperoni slices
Cheese for topping
1 small can tomato paste
Pinch of oregano
¼ teaspoon olive oil

Set aside ¼ cup mozzarella cheese. Mix remaining ingredients together in a mixing bowl. Place mini-waffle maker on a plate to avoid a messy clean-up, in case the mixture spills out of the sides. Plug in the waffle maker and spray it with oil. When the waffle maker is hot, sprinkle ¼ cup of cheese on the griddle. When the cheese is melted, spoon a thin layer of the mixture over the griddle, covering it. Close the top and allow the chaffle to cook about 4 minutes. When the chaffle is golden brown in color and crispy around the edges, remove it carefully. (To use the chaffles as sandwich buns, omit the remaining steps and add sandwich ingredients.)

Pizza sauce: in a small mixing bowl, combine the tomato paste, olive oil, and a pinch of oregano. Spoon pizza sauce onto the top of the chaffle to taste. Add cheese and cover with pepperoni slices. Place under an oven broiler and heat until cheese is melted. Enjoy!

Menus

DAY 1

Breakfast
2 large eggs, scrambled (2 grams carbs)
3 slices turkey bacon (1g)
¼ cup blueberries (5.4g)

Snack
Cheddar cheese stick (1g)

Lunch
Grilled chicken breast (0g)
Large salad (2 cups iceberg lettuce, 2g; ½ medium avocado, 6.5g; ½ cup of cherry tomatoes, 3g; bacon crumbles, 0g; and ¼ cup cheese, 2g; total: 13.5g)

Snack
100-calorie pack of almonds (3g)

Dinner
Baked salmon (1 filet) with dry seasoning of choice (1g)
Grilled asparagus, six spears (3g)
Side salad (lettuce, tomato, cucumber) with ranch, blue cheese, or balsamic vinaigrette dressing (6g)

DAY 2

Breakfast
Ham, cheese, and spinach frittata (0 grams carbs)
2 muffins (2g)
½ cup strawberries (6g)

Snack
Premier protein shake (3g)

Lunch
Medium beefsteak tomato (5g)
stuffed with tuna salad (canned tuna, mayonnaise, 2 hard-boiled eggs, pickled relish) (6g)
2 dill pickle spears (2g)

Snack
3 celery sticks (0g)
1 tablespoon peanut butter (4g)

Dinner
Air-fried, baked, or grilled chicken wings (0g)
Sweet Heat dry rub on the chicken (1g)
Baked zucchini fries (1 zucchini) (7g)

DAY 3

Breakfast
Two hard-boiled eggs (1.2 grams carbs)
3 slices bacon (0g)
½ cup chopped honey dew melon (6g)

Snack
1 stick of string cheese (0g)

Lunch
Grilled salmon (0g)
Caesar salad (2 cups Romaine lettuce, parmesan cheese, no croutons) (10g)
Caesar salad dressing (2g)

Snack
Bag of pork skins/Chicharrones (0g) or
11 green olives (1g)

Dinner
Grilled chicken breast (0g)
1 cup green beans with slivered almonds (7g)
½ medium baked sweet potato (20g)

DAY 4

Breakfast
Cheese omelet (4 grams carbs)
½ avocado, sliced (6.5g)

Snack
Homemade low-carb trail mix (5g)

Lunch
Bacon cheeseburger on lettuce wrap (3g)
3 tomato slices (3g)

Snack
Quest protein chips (5g)
or homemade kale chips, 1 cup (6g)

Dinner
Baked Cod (0g)
1 cup mashed cauliflower with sour cream and cheese (4g)
½ cup steamed broccoli (3g)

DAY 5

Breakfast

Sausage sandwich with chaffles (2 sausage patties between two savory chaffles) (1 gram carbs)
½ cup chopped honey dew melon (6g)

Snack

Cheese stick (1g)

Lunch

2 slices Keto pizza (cheese crust with meats of choice) (10g)
Side salad with ranch or balsamic vinaigrette dressing (1 cup iceberg lettuce with ½ cup cherry tomatoes) (4g)

Snack

Quest protein chips, tortilla-style, with 2 tablespoons cheese dip (8g)

Dinner

Grilled fish (tilapia, catfish, etc.) (0g)
1 cup egg salad on lettuce (3g)
½ cup mixed vegetables (6g)

DAY 6

Breakfast

Keto pancakes (2.5 grams carbs)
Bacon (0g)

Snack

Large hard-boiled egg (1g)

Lunch
Chicken salad (2.5g)
on 3 Romaine lettuce boats (3g)
3 Roma tomato slices (3g)
2 dill pickle spears (2g)

Snack
1 tablespoon dark chocolate morsels (8g)

Dinner
Low-carb enchiladas, 1 cup (4g)
½ cup pico de gallo (3g)
Guacamole, ¼ cup (5g)
Keto Spanish rice, ½ cup (5.5g)

DAY 7

Breakfast
Chaffles, two (1 gram carbs)
Mrs. Butterworth's sugar-free syrup, ¼ cup (4g)
Bacon (0g)

Snack
Turkey rolled around slice of cheese (2g)

Lunch
Bowl of no-beans chili (2 cups) (8g)
with shredded Mexican cheese (0g)
Sour cream (1g)
Side salad (1 cup lettuce and tomatoes) (5g)
Salad dressing (2g)

Snack
Whisps Cheese Crisps (1g)

Dinner
Baked turkey breast with gravy (3g)
Cauliflower rice, 1 cup (3g)
Green bean casserole, ¼ cup (7g)

DAY 8

Breakfast
Breakfast bowl with 2 eggs, sausage, bacon, green and red peppers, onions, and cheese (5 grams carbs)

Snack
Sugar-free candied pecans, ¼ cup (6g)

Lunch
Grilled shrimp (0g)
over mixed greens salad (6g)

Snack
Large hard-boiled egg (1g)

Dinner
Rotisserie chicken (0g)
Braised cabbage, ½ cup (7g)

DAY 9

Breakfast
Two-egg omelet with ¼ cup cooked spinach, green peppers, onion, and cheese (7 grams carbs)

Snack
Premier Protein Shake (5g)

Lunch
Turkey cheeseburger with chaffle buns, lettuce, and tomato (2g)
Keto coleslaw, 1 cup (2g)

Snack
Meat and cheese sticks (1g)

Dinner
Meatballs and low-carb marinara sauce (7g)
Spaghetti squash, ½ cup (5.5g)
Roasted brussels sprouts, ½ cup (4g)

Day 10

Breakfast
Low-carb breakfast pizza (chaffle crust, topped with breakfast sausage, bacon crumbles, peppers, onions, cheese) (5 grams carbs)

Snack
Pistachios, ½ cup (8g)

Lunch
Low-carb taco soup, 2 cups (10g)
1 tablespoon sour cream (1g)
Diced tomatoes (2g)

Snack
Whisps Cheese Crisps (1g)

Dinner
Chicken breast and ½ cup low-carb Alfredo sauce (4g)
Zoodles (zucchini noodles), 1 cup (2g)
Side Caesar salad (5g)

DAY 11

Breakfast
Breakfast wrap with two-egg "tortilla," sausage, cheese, avocado, tomato (7 grams carbs)

Snack
Dill pickle slices (0g)

Lunch
Grilled sirloin steak (0g)
1½ cups garden salad in a bag (3g)
½ cup cherry tomatoes (3g)

Snack
5 green olives stuffed with pimento (1g)

Dinner
Chicken Cacciatore, 1½ cups (6g)
Butternut squash noodles, ½ cup (11g)

DAY 12

Breakfast
Cottage cheese, ½ cup (4 grams carbs)
Blueberries (5.5 g)
Two slices of turkey bacon (0g)

Snack
Cherry tomatoes marinated in 1 tablespoon of balsamic vinaigrette (7g)

Lunch
Egg salad, 1 cup (3g)
Side salad (5g)

Snack
Mixed nuts, 1-ounce packet (8g)

Dinner
Beef stuffed zucchini boats, two (15 g)
Mixed vegetables, ½ cup (6g)

DAY 13

Breakfast
2 maple-flavored breakfast patties (4 grams carbs)
2 sliced hard-boiled eggs (2g)

Snack
½ cup raspberries with whipped cream (7g)

Lunch
Classic Cobb salad with grilled chicken, bacon, avocado, tomatoes, blue cheese crumbles, hard-boiled egg (11g)
Salad Dressing (2g)

Snack
Beef or turkey jerky (3g)

Dinner
Ham steak (2g)
½ medium sweet potato (13g)
1 cup collard greens (2g)

DAY 14

Breakfast
Spinach, mozzarella, and mushroom omelet (5 grams carbs)

Snack
Salami-cheese wrap (1g)

Lunch
3 BLT (bacon, lettuce, tomato) wraps (6g)
Low-carb beef vegetable soup, 1 cup (6g)

Snack
Hummus, 2 tablespoons (5g)
Celery sticks (0g)

Dinner
Stuffed bell peppers with ground beef (or turkey) and shrimp, two halves (8g)
Steamed cabbage (3g)
Cauliflower "mac" and cheese (7g)

5-Day Low-Carb Mediterranean Meal Guide

DAY 1

Breakfast
Greek yogurt with ¼ cup of strawberries (10 grams carbs)

Snack
¼ Blueberries (5 g)

Lunch
Tuna salad, dressed in olive oil (10g)

Dinner
Mediterranean low-carb lasagna (10g)

DAY 2

Breakfast
Omelet with veggies, tomatoes, and onions, cooked in olive oil
¼ cup raspberries (10 grams carbs)

Snack
½ cup of nuts (4g)

Lunch

Mediterranean low-carb pizza, topped with cheese, veggies, and olives (12g)

Dinner

Cod with garlic and black pepper (0g)

1 cup of arugula with cherry tomatoes, cucumber, and feta cheese, dressed in olive oil (4g)

DAY 3

Breakfast

2 fried egg with grilled tomatoes (5 grams carbs)

Snack

1 diced avocado (15g)

Lunch

2 cups of steamed spinach and 1 boiled artichoke mixed with lemon juice and herbs, olive oil, garlic powder, and salt (16g)

Dinner

½ cup zucchini pasta with low-carb spaghetti sauce, olive oil, and grilled vegetables with 1 tablespoon of Parmesan cheese (15g)

DAY 4

Breakfast

1 cup of Greek yogurt mixed with shredded almonds and blueberries (15 grams carbs)

Snack

Lox with cream cheese (you can have it over a Chaffle) (5g)

Lunch

2 cups of mixed greens with tomato and cucumber topped with roasted chicken, dressed with olive oil and lemon juice (6g)

Dinner

Oven-roasted vegetable (artichoke, zucchini, eggplant, tomato), tossed in olive oil and herbs with ¼ cup of whole-grain couscous (20g)

DAY 5

Breakfast

Spinach and feta frittata (5 grams carbs)

Snack

Hummus with celery (2g)

Lunch

Greek salad dressed in olive oil (10g)

Dinner

Broiled salmon with lemon, mustard, and herbs
Side salad with olive oil (2g)

Acknowledgements

No Guesswork was born out of me wanting to help America get healthy. With all the misinformation out there, I wanted to put together a body of work that got rid of all the confusion about diet and exercise. I truly want to take the guesswork out of healthy living. I hope this book achieves that. I put a lot of hard work and long hours into this book. The sacrifice was enormous. But this subject is my passion, and I would gladly do it all over again, if needed. I am so proud of this book, and I will carry it like a badge of honor. But it wouldn't have been possible without the help from some amazing people that God put in my life to help my vision come to pass. And I would like to acknowledge them here.

First and foremost, I would like to thank Lisa Frazier Page, who helped me write this book. Lisa, thank you so much. You were like my personal trainer, who made sure I showed up every day to do my daily workout for this book. As much passion as you know I have for this book and this topic, I don't know if I would have been able to have the stamina to finish it in the time that we did if you weren't there helping in this process. Your writing capability, patience and insight are one of a kind, and I am fortunate to have had you as a partner in writing this book. Your encouragement and wisdom helped me become a better writer and allowed me to take what was in my head and put it on paper. Thank you.

Anne Cole Norman, thanks for doing a wonderful job editing this book. You were such a critical piece to this book. Your skill and encouragement were invaluable.

I'd like to thank Stephanie for an awesome cover design and David Provolo for the wonderful interior design that made this book so great.

Thanks to all of my patients who have trusted me to guide them on this journey and taught me so much along the way. I offer a special thanks to Sharon Joachim and William "Bill" Reeves for allowing me to share their stories in this book. Sharon, your story encouraged me to start on this journey to learn as much as I could to help patients get to a healthier weight. Your determination, dedication and discipline, were admirable traits that I rarely saw with such consistency. Your grace and calming demeanor are inspiring.

Bill, thank you for believing in the process and showing up week after week. Even though the science was clear to me, your journey was a shining example of the effectiveness of NGW. Your determination, dedication, and discipline allowed you to lose hundreds of pounds through this program, and your success is a testament to all those who struggle with their weight. You are truly a beckon of hope. I hope both of you get to tell your full stories one day soon.

Joann Davis, thank you for believing in me and believing in us (The Three Doctors) from the very beginning of our journey as young adults. Without you, I wouldn't even be here to write this book. Thanks for your encouragement and for giving me the confidence to pursue this endeavor. You are truly one special lady.

Dr. George Jenkins and Dr. Sampson Davis, my two brothers from another mother, we are The Three Doctors! Trying to be superheroes. And we have been out here for decades trying to inspire the next generation of children to help make this world a better place. I love you, brothers. Our motto remains, "Our Children Cannot Aspire To Be What They Cannot See." And The Three Doctors have been out here in the world so that they can see us.

Nneka, thank you for being my rock and being there for me when I was finishing up the book. I Love you.

I'd like to thank my family: My mom, Arlene Hunt, and my sisters, Mecca, Daaimah and Quamara. To all my aunts, uncles, nieces/nephews and cousins, thank you for your love and support. I'd like to thank my grandmother, Winnie Jones, and also my grandmother, Ellen Bradley, who is looking out for me from heaven. And finally, I'd like to thank my dad, Alim, who is looking down on me and saying, "That's my boy!" There are so many more family members and friends who I love and who have loved and supported me, too many to name, but I just want to say thank you to them, as well.

Notes

Introduction

"Obesity is epidemic": Craig M. Hales, Margaret D. Carroll, Cheryl D. Fryar, and Cynthia L. Ogden, "Prevalence of Obesity and severe obesity among adults: United States, 2017-2018. *NCHS Data Brief*, no. 360. (February 2020)

"The prevalence of obesity in children": Craig M. Hales, Margaret D. Carroll, Cheryl D. Fryar, and Cynthia L. Ogden, "Prevalence of obesity among adults and youth: United States, 2015–2016." *NCHS Data Brief*, no 288. (October 2017)

Chapter 1

"Sharon was a 45-year-old wife and mother": Personal interview, shared with the patient's permission

"A nationwide study of attitudes and behaviors": Lee M. Kaplan et al, "Perceptions of Barriers to Effective Obesity Care: Results from the National ACTION Study," *Obesity*, (October 2017), https://doi.org/10.1002/oby.22054

"Dr. Westman had written a book": Dr. Eric Westman, *A Low Carbohydrate, Ketogenic Diet Manual: No Sugar, No Starch Diet* (CreateSpace Independent Publishing Platform, 2013)

"Carbs make up about half of the typical American diet": FastStats Homepage, CDC/National Center for Health Statistics, last reviewed May 3, 2017, https://www.cdc.gov/nchs/fastats/diet.htm

"a documentary called *Fed Up*": Stephanie Soechtig, Director, *Fed Up* (Jan. 19, 2014; Park City, Utah: Atlas Films, May 9, 2014), Documentary Film

"In the 1980s, almost no kids had Type 2 diabetes": "Prevent Type 2 Diabetes In Kids," Centers for Disease Control and Prevention, last updated June 29, 2017, https://www.cdc.gov/features/prevent-diabetes-kids/index.html

"But by 2015, a total of 193,000 children and adolescents younger than 20 were diagnosed with diabetes": "National Diabetes Statistics Report, 2017," Centers for Disease Control and Prevention, last reviewed March 6, 2018, https://www.cdc.gov/diabetes/data/statistics-report/index.html

"60 percent of packaged foods and drinks purchased from American grocery stores": Margot Sanger-Katz, "You'd Be Surprised at How Many Foods Contain Added Sugar," *New York Times,* May 21, 2016, https://www.nytimes.com/2016/05/22/upshot/it-isnt-easy-to-figure-out-which-foods-contain-sugar.html

"sugar is even more addictive than cocaine": Magalie Lenoir, Fuschia Serre, Lauriane Cantin, Serge H. Ahmed, "Intense sweetness surpasses cocaine reward," PLOS One, published Aug. 1, 2007, https://doi.org/10.1371/journal.pone.0000698

"In the late 1970s during U.S. Senate hearings for the first-ever dietary guidelines for American people": Gary Taubes, *Good Calories, Bad Calories: Challenging the Conventional Wisdom on Diet, Weight Control, and Disease* (New York: Albert Knopf, 2007)

"71 percent of all Americans are either overweight or obese": "Normal Weight, Overweight, and Obesity Among Adults Age 20 and Over, By Selected Characteristics: United States, Selected Years 1988-1994 through 2013-2016," Table 26, Centers for Disease Control and Prevention, accessed Dec. 3, 2019, https://www.cdc.gov/nchs/data/hus/2018/026.pdf

"Americans' attempts to lose weight have declined over time": Kassandra R. Snook et al., "Change in Percentages of Adults With Overweight or Obesity Trying to Lose Weight, 1988-2014," *JAMA* 317, no. 9 (March 1, 2017): 971–973, https://doi.org/10.1001/jama.2016.20036

"A group of researchers from the Johns Hopkins": Youfa Wang et al, "Will All Americans Become Overweight or Obese? Estimating the Progression and Cost of the U.S. Obesity Epidemic." *Obesity* 16, no. 10 (October 2008): 2323-30, https://doi.org/10.1038/oby.2008.351

Chapter 2

"After watching a documentary about processed food and meat": Kip Andersen, Keegan Kuhn, Directors, (2017). *What the Health,* (March 7, 2017); New York: A.U.M. Films & Media, March 7, 2017, Documentary Film

"In fact, a stack of evidence has shown the opposite: that high-carb intake, such as the consumption of sugary beverages, is directly associated with heart disease": Lindsay J. Collin et al, "Association of Sugary Beverage Consumption With Mortality Risk in US Adults: A Secondary Analysis of Data From the REGARDS Study," *JAMA Network Open 2*, no. 5 (May 17, 2019): e193121, https://doi.org/10.1001/jamanetworkopen.2019.3121

"High-carb intake can also lead to pre-diabetes": Collin et al, "Association of Sugary Beverage Consumption, **"As a matter of fact, a high-carb diet leads to a four-fold increase in the rate of cardiovascular disease with diabetes":** American Heart Association, last reviewed August 30, 2015, https://www.heart.org/en/health-topics/diabetes/why-diabetes-matters/cardiovascular-disease—diabetes

"The average calorie intake in the 1970s": Drew Desilver, "What's On Your Table? How America's Diet Has Changed Over The Decades," Pew Research Center, December 13, 2016, https://www.pewresearch.org/fact-tank/2016/12/13/whats-on-your-table-how-americas-diet-has-changed-over-the-decades/

"It's hard to say whether the low-fat diet was the cause of the stroke": Christopher E. Ramsden et al, "Re-evaluation Of the Traditional Diet-Heart Hypothesis: Analysis of Recovered Data from Minnesota Coronary Experiment (1968-73)," *BMJ* 353 (April 12, 2016): i1246 *https://doi.org/10.1136/bmj.i1246*

"The combined data also showed that saturated fat may even help to prevent strokes": Patty W. Siri-Tarino, Qi Sun, Frank B Hu, and Ronald M Krauss, "Meta-analysis Of Prospective Cohort Studies Evaluating the Association of Saturated Fat with Cardiovascular Disease," *The American Journal of Clinical Nutrition* 91, no. 3, (March 2010): 535–546, https://doi.org/10.3945/ajcn.2009.27725

"Those reports were based on a 1973 study": Hershel Jick et al, "Coffee and Myocardial Infarction." *New England Journal of Medicine* 289 (July 12, 1973):63-67, https://www.nejm.org/doi/full/10.1056/NEJM197307122890203

"A number of meta-analysis studies have shown the same": Nutrition Coalition, "The Disputed Science on Saturated Fats," accessed Nov. 30, 2019, https://www.nutritioncoalition.us/saturated-fats-do-they-cause-heart-disease/

"when your body becomes insulin resistant it goes in this order": Lorraine P Turcotte, Jonathan S Fisher, "Skeletal Muscle Insulin Resistance: Roles of Fatty Acid Metabolism and Exercise," *Physical Therapy* 88, no. 11 (November 1, 2008): 1279–1296, https://doi.org/10.2522/ptj.20080018

"So when your other cells are becoming resistant": Ralph A. DeFronzo, Devjit Tripathy, "Skeletal Muscle Insulin Resistance Is the Primary Defect in Type 2 Diabetes," *Diabetes Care* 32, (suppl 2) (November 2009): S157-S163, https://doi.org/10.2337/dc09-S302

"Let's start with making the case that in general": Park Y, Nam S, Yi HJ, Hong HJ, Lee M. "Dietary n-3 polyunsaturated fatty acids increase oxidative stress in rats with intracerebral hemorrhagic stroke", *Nutrition Research* 29 (11) (November 2009) https://www.ncbi.nlm.nih.gov/pubmed/19932870
Yerushalmy J, Hilleboe H. "Fat in the diet and mortality from heart disease", figure 2 (vascular lesions affecting the central nervous system), *New York State Journal of Medicine* 57 (14) (July 1957) https://www.ncbi.nlm.nih.gov/pubmed/13441073
DiNoclantonio J. "The cardiometabolic consequences of replacing saturated fats with carbohydrates or omega-6 polyunsaturated fats: Do the dietary guidelines have it wrong?" *BMJ Open Heart* (March 5, 2014) https://openheart.bmj.com/content/1/1e000032

Chapter 3

"The majority of people who lose weight": Rudolph L. Leibel et al., "Biologic Responses to Weight Loss and Weight Regain: Report From an American Diabetes Association Research Symposium," *Diabetes* 64, no.7 (July 2015): 2299-2309, https://doi.org/10.2337/db15-0004

"Of all the three macronutrients": Wendy A.M. Blom et al., "Effect of a high-protein breakfast on the postprandial ghrelin response," *The American Journal Of Clinical Nutrition* 83, no. 2 (February 1, 2006): 211-220, https://doi.org/10.1093/ajcn/83.2.211

"It's a powerful driver of cravings": Nicole M. Avena, Pedro Rada, Bartley G. Hoebel, "Evidence For Sugar Addiction: Behavioral and Neurochemical Effects of Intermittent, Excessive Sugar Intake," *Neuroscience & Biobehavioral Reviews* 32, no.1 (2008): 20-39, https://doi.org/10.1016/j.neubiorev.2007.04.019

"As a result, many people who get the Lap Band": "Lap Band Success Rate: What You Need To Know," Obesity News Today, accessed January 21, 2020, https://obesitynewstoday.com/lap-band-success-rate/

"So all the hype about leptin was a bust": University of Cincinnati Academic Health Center, "Obesity Research Finds Leptin Hormone Isn't the Overeating Culprit," *ScienceDaily*, accessed December 12, 2019, www.sciencedaily.com/releases/2015/05/150518145437.htm

"80 percent of the people who lose weight gain it back": University of Melbourne, "Obese People Regain Weight After Dieting Due to Hormones, Australian study finds," *ScienceDaily*, 31 October 31, 2011, www.sciencedaily.com/releases/2011/10/111028142504.htm

"A study by Fabrizio Benedetti": Fabrizio Benedetti, Elisa Carlino, and Antonella Pollo, "How Placebos Change the Patient's Brain." *Neuropsychopharmacology* 36, no. 1 (June 30, 2010): 339–354, https://doi.org/10.1038/npp.2010.81

"Dr. Alia Crum, a psychologist from Stanford University": Alia J. Crum, Ellen J. Langer, "Mind-set Matters: Exercise and the Placebo Effect," *Psychological Science* 18, no. 2 (February 1, 2007): 165-171. https://doi.org/10.1111/j.1467-9280.2007.01867.x

"Dr. Crum conducted a similar study with two groups of university students": Alia J. Crum, William R. Corbin, Kelly D. Brownell, Peter Salovey, "Mind Over Milkshakes: Mindsets, Not Just Nutrients, Determine Ghrelin Response," *Health Psychology* 30, no. 4 (July 2011): 424-4299; https://doi.org/10.1037/a0023467

"Author Daniel Coyle explores this phenomenon": Daniel Coyle, *The Talent Code: Greatness Isn't Born. It's Grown* (Arrow Books Ltd, 2010)

"Writer James Clear, who studies habits": James Clear, *Atomic Habits: An Easy & Proven Way to Build Good Habits & Break Bad Ones* (Avery, 2018)

"One such researcher was Phillippa Lally": Phillippa Lally, Cornelia H. M. van Jaarsveld,
Henry W. W. Potts, Jane Wardle, "How Are Habits Formed: Modeling Habit formation in the Real World." *European Journal of Social Psychology* (July 16, 2009), https://doi.org/10.1002/ejsp.674

"Professor Wendy Wood, who teaches psychology": Wendy Wood, *Good Habits, Bad Habits: The Science of Making Positive Changes That Stick* (Farrar, Straus and Giroux, 2019)

"The thoughtful intentional mind is easily derailed.": Society for Personality and Social Psychology, "How We Form Habits, Change Existing Ones," *ScienceDaily* (August 8, 2014), www.sciencedaily.com/releases/2014/08/140808111931.htm

"Be mindful when you eat": Megrette Fletcher, "What is Mindful Eating? Hint: It's Not Just About Chewing Your Food For a Long Time," *mindful, healthy mind, healthy life* (January 26, 2016), https://www.mindful.org/what-is-mindful-eating/

Chapter 5

"Between 5 percent and 10 percent is the amount of weight loss needed": Donald A. Williamson, George A. Bray, Donna H. Ryan, *Obesity* 23, no. 12 (December 2015): 2319-2320, https://doi.org/10.1002/oby.21358

"That is the amount of weight that you need to lose to see improvements": Damon L. Swift et al., "Effects of Clinically Significant Weight Loss With Exercise Training on Insulin Resistance and Cardiometabolic Adaptations." *Obesity* 24, no. 4: 812–819, https://doi.org/10.1002/oby.21404

"legislation from the Affordable Care Act of 2010": U.S. Food and Drug Administration, updated March 26, 2018, https://www.fda.gov/about-fda/economic-impact-analyses-fda-regulations/summary-food-labeling-nutrition-labeling-standard-menu-items-restaurants-and-similar-retail-food

"The HMS predicts how well you will do": Hunt R., Obesity Week 2018 "Validation of the Hunt Motivational Scale" https://2018.obesityweek.com/abstract/validation-of-the-hunt-motivational-scale/

Chapter 6

"Medical doctors prescribe ketogenic diets": Roberto R. Caraballo et al., "Long-term Follow-up of the Ketogenic Diet for Refractory Epilepsy: Multicenter Argentinean Experience in 216 Pediatric Patients," *Seizure* 20, no. 8 (October 2011):640-645, https://doi.org/10.1016/j.seizure.2011.06.009

"The medical truth is you don't need to eat carbs to survive": Anssi H. Manninen, "Metabolic Effects of the Very-Low-Carbohydrate Diets: Misunderstood "Villains" Of Human Metabolism," *Journal of the International Society of Sports Nutrition* 1, no. 7 (Dec. 10, 2004): 7–11. https://doi.org/10.1186/1550-2783-1-2-7

"The body needs about 110 to 140 grams of carbs to fuel your brain": Food and Nutrition Board, Institute of Medicine of the National Academies, *Dietary Reference Intakes For Energy, Carbohydrate, Fiber, Fat, Fatty Acids, Cholesterol, Protein, and Amino Acids* (Washington, D.C.: National Academies Press, 2005), 277-278. https://www.nal.usda.gov/sites/default/files/fnic_uploads/energy_full_report.pdf

"a man's body makes about 250 grams of carbs per day": Food and Nutrition Board, 276-277

"your brain can use ketones for about 80 percent of the energy": Food and Nutrition Board, 277-278

"It is well documented that a low-carb ketogenic diet raises good cholesterol": William S. Yancy, Jr. et al, "A Low-Carbohydrate, Ketogenic Diet versus a Low-Fat Diet To Treat Obesity and Hyperlipidemia: A Randomized, Controlled Trial," *Annals Of Internal Medicine* 140, no. 10 (May 18, 2004): 769-777, https://annals.org/aim/fullarticle/717451/low-carbohydrate-ketogenic-diet-versus-low-fat-diet-treat-obesity

"There are prospective randomized, long-term (greater than a year) studies": Nassib Bezerra Bueno et al., "Very-Low-Carbohydrate Ketogenic Diet v. Low-fat Diet for Long-term Weight Loss: A Meta-Analysis of Randomised Controlled Trials," *British Journal of Nutrition* 110, no. 7 (May 7, 2013): 1178-1187. https://doi.org/10.1017/S0007114513000548
"Is the study of them not long-term enough": Caraballo et al, "Long-term follow-up," 640-645

"And some studies even showed that people on high-carb diets have increased mortality": Mahshid Dehghan et al., "Associations of Fats and Carbohydrate Intake With Cardiovascular Disease and Mortality in 18 Countries From Five Continents (PURE): A Prospective Cohort Study," *The Lancet* 390, no. 10107 (November 4,2017): 2050-2062, https://doi.org/10.1016/S0140-6736(17)32252-3. Estruch R, et al., "Primary Prevention of Cardiovascular Disease with a Mediterranean Diet (PREDIMED)", *The New England Journal of Medicine* 2013 (368: 1279-1290) (April 4, 2013)

"the Look Ahead trial...had to be stopped early": The Look AHEAD Research Group, "Cardiovascular Effects of Intensive Lifestyle Intervention in Type 2 Diabetes," *New England Journal of Medicine* 369 (July 11, 2013): 145-154, https://www.nejm.org/doi/full/10.1056/NEJMoa1212914

"Another trial, called the WHI study": Barbara V. Howard et al., "Low-Fat Dietary Pattern and Risk of Cardiovascular Disease: The Women's Health Initiative Randomized Controlled Dietary Modification Trial," *Journal of the American Medical Association* 295, no. 6 (February 8, 2006): 655–666, https://doi.org/10.1001/jama.295.6.655

"Yet another multi-million-dollar study, known as the Nurses Study": Michelle D. Holmes et al., "Association of Dietary Intake of Fat and Fatty Acids With Risk of Breast Cancer," *Journal of the American Medical Association* 281, no. 10 (March 10, 1999): 914-920, https://doi.org/10.1001/jama.281.10.914

"High sugar (i.e. diabetes/pre-diabetes/insulin resistance) puts you at risk for heart attacks and strokes": Centers for Disease Control and Prevention, "Diabetes, Heart Disease, and You," last updated Nov. 23, 2016, https://www.cdc.gov/features/diabetes-heart-disease/index.html
Haffner SM, Lehto S, Ronnemaa T, Pyoraia K, Laakso M., "Mortality from coronary heart disease in subjects with type 2 diabetes and in nondiabetic subjects with and without prior myocardial infarction." *New England Journal of Medicine* 339 (4) (July 23, 1998)

Umemura T, Kawamura T., "Effect of diabetes on stroke symptoms and mortality: Lessons from a recent large population-based cohort study." *Journal of Diabetes Investigation* 5 (1) (February 12, 2014)

"The absorption of the small percentage of unesterified": Wang L. "New insights into the genetic regulation of intestinal cholesterol absorption", *Gastroenterology Journal* 129 (2: 718-734) (August 2005)
https://www.gastrojournal.org/article/S0016-5085(04)02028-1/

Chapter 7

"Lori, a technology consultant": The patient's story is real, but her name was changed to protect her privacy

"Ellie, a patient of mine in her thirties who works as a busy office manager": The patient's story is real, but her name was changed to protect her privacy

"Studies say, that, too, is just a myth.": Jessica Brown, "Is Breakfast Really the Most Important Meal of the Day?" *BBC Future,* November 27, 2018, https://www.bbc.com/future/article/20181126-is-breakfast-good-for-your-health

"If you don't get the appropriate sleep": Sebastian M. Schmid et al, "A Single Night Of Sleep Deprivation Increases Ghrelin Levels and Feelings of Hunger in Normal-Weight Healthy Men," *Journal of Sleep Research* 17, no.3 (September 2008): 331-334. https://doi.org/10.1111/j.1365-2869.2008.00662.x

"Studies show that shift workers": Wiley, "Night Shift Work Linked To an Increased Risk of Obesity." *ScienceDaily*, accessed December 12, 2019, www.sciencedaily.com/releases/2017/10/171004084933.htm

"Stress also increases ghrelin": UT Southwestern Medical Center, "Hunger Hormone Increases During Stress, May Have Antidepressant Effect," *ScienceDaily*, www.sciencedaily.com/releases/2008/06/080615142252.htm

"In science, we call the energy you burn when you're not sleeping, eating, or working out in a gym Non-Exercise Activity Thermogenesis": James A. Levine, "Non-Exercise Activity Thermogenesis (NEAT)," *Best Practice & Research Clinical Endocrinology & Metabolism* 16, no. 4 (December 2002): 679-702, https://doi.org/10.1053/beem.2002.0227

Chapter 8

"With intermittent fasting, you alternate periods of eating and fasting,": Roger Collier, "Intermittent Fasting: The Science Of Going Without," *Canadian Medical Association Journal* 185, no. 9 (June 11, 2013); E363–E364. https://doi.org/10.1503/cmaj.109-4451

"Intermittent fasting is good because it works the same as a well-formulated low-carb diet; they both keep your insulin level low": Monique Tello, "Intermittent Fasting: Surprising Update," *Harvard Health Publishing*, Harvard Medical School, June 29, 2018. https://www.health.harvard.edu/blog/intermittent-fasting-surprising-update-2018062914156

Chapter 9

"When I first met William "Bill" Reeves, Jr.": Personal interview, shared with the patient's permission

"Since 2012, the FDA has approved four new weight loss drugs": "Prescription Medications to Treat Overweight and Obesity," National Institute of Diabetes and Digestive and Kidney Diseases, https://www.niddk.nih.gov/health-information/weight-management/prescription-medications-treat-overweight-obesity

"Interestingly, the sleeve was developed as a weight loss option by accident": David Benaiges et al., "Laparoscopic Sleeve Gastrectomy: More Than a Restrictive Bariatric Surgery Procedure?" *World Journal Of Gastroenterology* 21, no. 41 (Nov. 7, 2015): 11804–11814. https://www.ncbi.nlm.nih.gov/pmc/articles/PMC4631978/

"gastric bypass is still the most effective surgical procedure": David Arterburn et al., "Comparative Effectiveness and Safety of Bariatric Procedures for Weight Loss: A PCORnet Cohort Study," *Annals of Internal Medicine* 169, no. 11 (Dec. 4, 2018): 741–750. https://doi.org/10.7326/M17-2786

"A study done by Dr. Louis Aronne": Alpana P. Shukla, Radu G. Iliescu, Catherine E. Thomas, Louis J. Aronne, "Food Order Has a Significant Impact on Postprandial Glucose and Insulin Levels," *Diabetes Care*, 38, no.7 (July 2015): e98–e99. https://doi.org/10.2337/dc15-0429

Chapter 10

"Cara's goal was to lose 100 pounds": The patient's story is real, but her name was changed to protect her privacy

"A study of fourteen contestants who participated in the once wildly popular televised weight loss show": Erin Fothergill et al., *Obesity* 24, no. 8 (August 2016): 1612–1619, https://doi.org/10.1002/oby.21538

"I've got my life back,": Gina Kolata, "After 'The Biggest Loser,' Their Bodies Fought to Regain Weight," *New York Times Magazine,* May 2, 2016

"A study done by Dr. Michael Rosenbaum": Gina Kolata, "Short Answers to Hard Questions About Weight Loss." *New York Times,* May 4, 2016

"Likewise, a 2018 study by Dr. David Ludwig of Harvard University": Cara B. Ebbeling et al., "Effects of a Low Carbohydrate Diet on Energy Expenditure During Weight Loss Maintenance: Randomized Trial," *The BMJ* 363 (November 14, 2018): k4583, https://www.bmj.com/content/363/bmj.k4583

"One small study of 50 overweight or obese adults had them lose weight on a meal replacement diet": Priya Sumithran et al., "Long-term Persistence of Hormonal Adaptations to Weight Loss," *New England Journal of Medicine* 365 (October 27, 2011): 1597-1604 https://www.nejm.org/doi/full/10.1056/NEJMoa1105816

"Studies have shown the Mediterranean Diet is the best": Kris Gunnars, "5 Studies on The Mediterranean Diet - Does it Really Work?" retrieved from healthline.com, May 29, 2017. https://www.healthline.com/nutrition/5-studies-on-the-mediterra-nean-diet

"First there is something called The French Paradox"
The French Paradox: lessons for other countries
https://www.ncbi.nlm.nih.gov/pmc/articles/PMC1768013

"One thought was that the protection was because the French drank more red wine" Absorption of three wine-related polyphenols in three different matrices by healthy subjects
https://www.ncbi.nlm.nih.gov/pubmed/12554065

"This was shown in a re-analysis of data from fourteen of the countries..."
Food industry funding of nutrition research. The relevance of history for current debates

https://jamanetwork.com/journals/jamainternalmedicine/article-abstract/2548251
Dietary fats, Carbohydrates and Atherosclerotic Vascular disease
https://www.nejm.org/doi/full/10.1056/NEJM196708032770505

"His Seven Country Study..."
https://www.sevencountriesstudy.com/about-the-study/investigators/ancel-keys/

Permissions

CHAPTER 1

GENETICS PLAY A MAJOR ROLE IN OBESITY
Source: Borgjeson Acta Paediatrica May 1976. https://onlinelibrary.wiley.com/doi/abs/10.1111/j.1651-2227.1976.tb04887.x
Permission: Copyright Clearance Center

CHAPTER 2

A LOW-CARB DIET IS COLORFUL
Source and permission: pexels.com and istockphoto.com

DEGENERATIVE HEART DISEASE
Source: Journal of Mount Sinai 1953; 20 (2); 118-139.
Permission: Copyright Clearance Center

DRS. YERUSHALMY AND HILLEBOE: MORTALITY FROM ARTERIOSCLEROTIC AND DEGENERATIVE HEART DISEASE AND FAT CALORIES FROM 22 COUNTRIES IN MEN 55-59 YEARS OLD
Source: New York State Journal of Medicine July 15th 1957; 57 (14): 2343-54.
Permission: Medical Society of the State of New York.

SIDE BY SIDE COMPARISION: ANCEL KEYS GRAPH (ON LEFT- 6 COUNTRIES) AND YERUSHALMY AND HILLEBOE (ON RIGHT- 22 COUNTRIES)
Source: New York State Journal of Medicine July 15th 1957; 57 (14): 2343-54 and Journal of Mount Sinai 1953; 20 (2); 118-139.
Permission: Copyright Clearance Center and Medical Society of the State of New York

PREVALENCE OF OBESITY AMONG US ADULTS AGED 20-74
Source: NHANES. http://www.cdc.gov/nchs/data/hestat/obesity_adult_09_10/obesity_adult_09_10.html#table1
Permission: public domain

KWASHIORKOR
Source: CDC/ Robert S. Craig and Dr. Lyle Conrad
Permission: public domain

MARASMUS
Source: CDC/Don Eddins
Permission: public domain

MAASAI
Source and permission: istock.com.

BEER BELLY
Source and permission: istock.com.

CHAPTER 3

HUNGER GREMLIN, GHRELIN
Source and permission: istock.com.

GUT HORMONES PLAY A CRITICAL ROLE IN HUNGER AND SATIETY VIA THE APPETITE CENTER IN YOUR BRAIN
Source design: Dr. Hunt
Permission for images: pexels.com

TYPES OF BARIATRIC SURGERY
Source and Permission: istock.com

GHRELIN AND OTHER GUT HORMONES THAT HELP REGULATE YOUR THERMOSTAT (I.E. SET POINT)
Source design: Dr. Hunt
Permission: pexels.com

MOUSE PICTURE
Source and Permission: istock.com

YOUNG BOY WITH LEPTIN DEFICIENCY (ON LEFT) AND THEN AFTER WWTREATMENT (ON RIGHT)
Source: Source: Journal of Endocrinology 2014. https://joe.bioscientifica.com/view/journals/joe/223/1/T63.xml
Permission: Copyright Clearance Center

THE FAT CELL CAN CAUSE AND IS ASSOCIATED WITH MANY DIFFERENT MEDICAL CONDITIONS
Source Design: Dr. Hunt
Permission for image: pexels.com

CHAPTER 6

LOW CARB DIET
Permission: pexels.com and istockphoto.com

Chapter 10

NORMAL AND LOW CARB MEDITERRANEAN DIET
Source and Permission: pexels.com

Made in the USA
Columbia, SC
09 July 2020